LIVE DISEASE FREE

A Practical Guide to Health,
Healing, and Vitality

SATISH GIRIJA

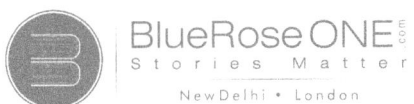

NewDelhi • London

BLUEROSE PUBLISHERS
India | U.K.

Copyright © Satish Kumar "Satish Girija" 2024

All rights reserved by author. No part of this publication may be reproduced, stored in a retrieval system or transmitted in any form or by any means, electronic, mechanical, photocopying, recording or otherwise, without the prior permission of the author. Although every precaution has been taken to verify the accuracy of the information contained herein, the publisher assumes no responsibility for any errors or omissions. No liability is assumed for damages that may result from the use of information contained within.

BlueRose Publishers takes no responsibility for any damages, losses, or liabilities that may arise from the use or misuse of the information, products, or services provided in this publication.

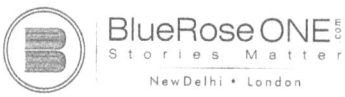

For permissions requests or inquiries regarding this publication, please contact:

BLUEROSE PUBLISHERS
www.BlueRoseONE.com
info@bluerosepublishers.com
+91 8882 898 898
+4407342408967

ISBN: 978-93-6452-304-2

Cover design: Shivam
Typesetting: Namrata Saini

First Edition: October 2024

Author's Note
(Preface)

I am of the age of 76 years old and work for 10 to 12 hours daily. I have almost no disease except few ageing problem. My heart, kidney, lungs, lever, thyroid, blood-pressure, eye-vision etc. everything is working perfectly. I get my comprehensive health-check-up every year on which basis I am writing this.

I have learnt by adopting healthy lifestyle in my own life, reading many books, talking to doctors specialized in different diseases, being a naturopathy practitioner, attending different seminars & meetings on health-issues that for any disease or health problems, our bad habits and unhealthy lifestyle, is mainly responsible. If you too analyse yourself deeply then certainly will recognise that for any disease, other than few unavoidable ageing problems, we ourselves are responsible for it.

Below mentioned are 12 healthy lifestyle in chapter one which can lead us to a disease-free life by sure. Even if you are having some disease, by following below mentioned lifestyle, you will get rid of them to a great extent. Described in other chapters about several diseases & its preventive measures and about how to keep our important organs of the body in good working condition, the tips given there, fully tally with what are mentioned in those 12 lifestyles for living disease free.

Adopting below mentioned lifestyle will cost you nothing, but only the determination, will-power and commitment. That will make your life disease-free, happy and peaceful. All the suggested lifestyles are doable and based on what I am already practicing, hence there is no doubt that you can also do it.

I have also given other important information in chapter 2 on our time-management & daily routine, about functioning of other organs & parts of body, precautionary measures to keep all of them in good working condition in Chapter 3 & 4, some food item I use in daily life (chapter 5) which medicinal properties keep us healthy and away from diseases Going thorough them and practicing the suggestions there, if every organ will function well and will be in good working condition, there will be no chances of any disease. If we shall be cautious about how disease attack us, then we can protect ourselves easily. Also, the food items, who can keep is healthy have been given in this book, so that we can make them a part of our daily diet. The timetable and the daily routine explained, can make your life well organized.

By changing a little in your daily routine, food-intake and adopting the healthy habits & lifestyle described in detail in this book and utilizing the useful information in other chapters smartly, I can assure you that you will live disease free, your medical expenses on doctors/ hospitals / medicines may come to zero. If you are at the old age, you can live a happy life. If you are in the working age, you can enjoy your work better, will not have to take any medical leave and can achieve your ambition & promotions very successfully. If you are a student, you will never miss your classes due to some disease and may have a better career & future.

I am very much thankful to website of Pixabay (https://pixabay.com/images/search/) and Freepik (https://www.freepik.com/free-photos-vectors/) providing royalty free images, used in this book. Also I am thankful to other sites on google which references used in this book mentioned in the pages where used.

I also extend my heartfelt thanks to Dr. Megha Sinha MBBS for going through the chapters on body organs and major diseases (chapter 3 and 4) and giving required suggestion incorporated, based on her experiences as a Medical Officer in a hospital in Hazaribagh-Jharkhand-India.

Please do write your comments, reading this book, practising the shared useful information in your life and its result. It will help me to further improve my experiences.

Hazaribagh, India   Satish Girija

September 2024   satishgirija@gmail.com

Contents

Chapter 1: The 12 Healthy Lifestyle for A Disease-Free Life..1

Chapter 2: Time management & A Sample Daily Routine/timetable to living Disease free.......................47

Chapter 3: Know about your important Organs of the body and how to keep them healthy to make you disease free...53

Chapter 4: Prevent some serious diseases to affect you..93

Chapter 5: Food Items that may be helpful to Keep you Disease Free..104

CHAPTER 1

The 12 Healthy Lifestyle for A Disease-Free Life

Change a little your Morning Routine (Blessings, Warm water, Ganesh Kriya, Splashing and Yoga)

1.1 When you open your eyes after the sleep in the morning, please first remember your God whom you worship and pray for the blessings to have your day meaningful, happy, healthy, and successful. For this you have not to go to your worship place but do it on your bed itself with your eyes closed, hands joined as in prayer and requesting for the blessings for the day. God is everywhere, you can remember & worship from anywhere.

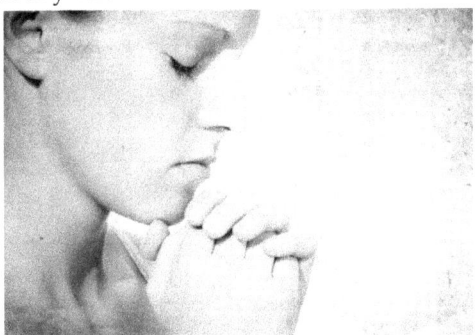

1.2 When you get-up, wish your family members, saying "good morning" (in your own family language) with a smile.

These both will give a peace and pleasure to your mind. Mind is very much linked with the health of your body and soul.

1.3 Start then the day drinking 2 glasses of warm water in the early morning and go for the toilet on time.

It is a proverb that "early to bed and early to rise- makes a person healthy, wealthy and wise". Try to get early to bed and rise early before the sunrise.

The practice of drinking warm water in the early morning empty stomach, will save you from many types of diseases. If possible, you can take a fresh lemon in hot water with a little rock salt and a pinch of black pepper powder. Lemonade and black pepper are helpful in increasing vitality or immunity.

1.4 After drinking warm water, please have some walk. It will accelerate the pressure for toilet.

Practice the habit of going to toilet at the same /fixed time every day in the morning, even if there is no stool for a few days in the beginning, but gradually you will start getting used to it and you will feel the pressure yourself at that time.

1.5 Then in the toilet practice Ganesh Kriya & Ashwini Mudra. Indian Ayurveda is one of the most scientific health manual, based on years of experimentation and results. By adopting Ganesh Kriya and Ashwini Mudra described in it, in our daily life, we will get rid of haemorrhoids or piles forever (a very common disease now-a-days), constipation, gastric and bowel diseases. By this you will experience lightness in our body and wonderful radiance on the face.

Ganesh-kriya is a process that helps to eliminate common complaints like partial or dissatisfying bowel evacuation, hard stools, erratic, difficult or painful bowel motions, constipation and forceful evacuation etc. Nevertheless, anyone can perform this kriya to experience its usefulness.

For Ganesh-kriya, while going to toilet, lubricate the forefinger of your left hand with some castor oil, ghee or sesame oil or in the toilet wet your middle figure with water. Then apply this lubricated/watery finger inside the anus very slowly and rotate it clockwise & anticlockwise for 4-5 times with a little pressure. Remember nails of that finger should be well cut. Then with that finger, take out and clean the solid substances or faeces stuck on the inner walls of anus. Generally, we clean our anus after defecation only from outside, while cleaning from inside & outside both are equally important, which we never do in general practice and get affected with many diseases like piles, gastric, constipation etc. because most of the time faeces remain inside the anus and get rotten or decomposed creating bad-gas, piles, constipation and diseases overtime.

By Ganesh Kriya, the sticking faeces and toxic elements in the intestine or inner part of anus, come out, get cleaned, making us fresh and saving us from many diseases. If inner anus not cleared after toilet, piles and many other disease will attack.

It is my firm believe that adopting Gansh Kriya by all, we can make the world "piles disease free", while piles at present is a very common disease.

1.6 After Ganesh Kriya, you do Ashwini Mudra. Ashwini means Horse - the symbol of power. One of the secrets of the strength and agility in the horse is Ashwini mudra. If you have ever noticed that after passing urine, the horse repeatedly contracts and loosens its anus. In Ashwini mudra, we have to copy this posture of horse. Contract and relax the anal muscles in a manner just like the horse does while passing excreta. Repeat the contraction-relaxation cycle 10 to 12 times. This is called as Ashwini Mudra.

In this era of fast food, it is very common to eat spicy, oily, packaged and dry food items. This and the irregular eating timings cause a stress on the digestive system. Many laxatives and purgatives are being advertised and sold claiming permanent relief from this problem. However, none of these medicine can strengthen the digestive system from within. The above mentioned kriyas are most useful, since they are in unison with nature's modus operandi.

Ashwini Mudra can be performed anywhere and at any time of the day. There is no need to allocate specific time for it.

Special Instruction: Ganesh Kriya and Ashwini mudra is not to be performed in case the anus is swollen due to piles or by other reason and if there is pain or cracks in that area.

Some Benefits of doing Ganesh Kriya and Ashwini Mudra-

- By Ganesh Kriya, the bad particles/faeces stuck inside anus, and toxic elements of the intestine are cleared.
- This action is beneficial to get rid of haemorrhoids or piles because the birth of haemorrhoids disease is due to the sticking of the remained stool or faeces in the intestine/anus and not cleaned out, which after few days get rotten/decomposed and create germs causing many diseases including piles. Therefore, those who never want to have haemorrhoids in their life should practice Ganesh Kriya. It should be done every day.
- By doing Ganesh Kriya, the problem of constipation is also removed, which is the main cause of many diseases.
- Due to the clearing of the stomach and the removal of constipation, there is a brightness on the face and the radiance increases.
- These exercise in the toilet strengthens and improves flexibility of muscles and blood vessels in the anus area. No other exercise can achieve this.
- Sluggishness of the organs diminishes, and one becomes swift and energetic like a horse.
- Piles and gas trouble may be eliminated for ever in one's life

- Listlessness and depression vanish, and confidence is generated.
- There is a lot of materials on these topics on Google or YouTube. For full details, please get more information and videos on Google or YouTube.

1.7 Then have your teeth brushed and the bath. Remember, as important as it is to brush your teeth in the morning, it is more important to brush your teeth before sleeping at night, because our mouth remains closed at night, due to which any food particles inside it get rotten and cause bad smell and gum-disease, cavity etc. Therefore, brush your teeth early morning as well as before going to bed at night. Many people brush their teeth after every eating. This habit is very good.

Rinse your mouth with enough water thoroughly after the teeth-brush and also after every eating or meal so that the food particles stuck in the teeth and gums dissolve and come out. With this practice you can stay safe from teeth and gum diseases.

For strengthening your teeth and gums, eat nuts, carrot, cucumber, apple, onion etc. daily cutting them with teeth, which makes an exercise for gums & teeth.

1.8 For keeping both eyes free from disease (a preventive tool) and better vision, one of the very easy and daily practice is splashing normal cold fresh & clean water in both the eyes keeping them open after every mouthwash, having your mouth full of water. I am practicing it daily and at the age of 76 years, my vision in both the eyes is 6/6- a normal person has.

1.9 Then have some exercise suitable to you for 15 to 20 minutes. Physical exercise is a must to remain healthy and disease free. Due to modern scientific development, our lifestyle has changed a lot, and most of us have not to do physical exercise and only spend our days on sitting. But to make every part of our body fit, functioning and free from any health problem, we have to keep them in good working condition by some simple physical exercises suitable to our age. By the physical exercise, I do not mean by any manual labour, but I mean to say walking, jogging, running, asanas & yoga, gym, swimming, playing out-door games etc. making every part of your body stimulated to remain fit.

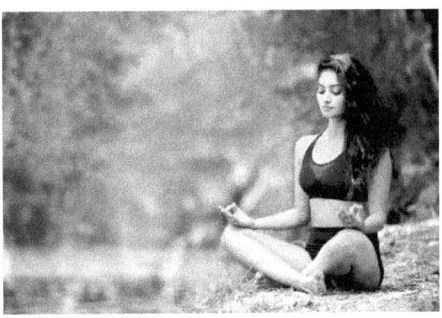

Doing 15-20 minutes (or more if time is available to you) of yoga-exercise or jogging-walking or in the evening playing badminton/cricket/tennis etc. any out-door games is very necessary to stay healthy & fit. In a 24-hour day, definitely take out 20to 30 minutes for yoga, asanas and physical exercises.

There is a lot of information available about yoga and asanas in books, television or internet or YouTube or google. Select yoga /asanas as per your interest and age or by consulting a yoga teacher and do them daily for 15-20 minutes.

It is very beneficial for children and youth to run on green grass early in the morning or in the evening. Girls and boys can also exercise by going to the gym. But instead of 'gym', it is better to do yoga, asanas and morning and evening walking, jogging, running, playing out-door games, swimming, or exercise.

Adults and older people should practice walking two to three kilometres outside in the morning or evening after some asana or yoga.

In view of the danger of Corona and other virus diseases, use a mask whenever you go out. The mask should be clean and completely cover the mouth and nose. Also maintain personal distance. By wearing a mask, personal distance and washing hands with soap from time to time, you can avoid the danger of corona or other viruses to a great extent. Therefore, take the above precautions while walking outside in the park

2.The Break-fast
(No Cooked Food in Breakfast)

The breakfast literally means "breaking the fast". Whenever we break the fast, we take juice, fruits and light foods. Same practice has to be adopted for our daily breakfast too. Do not take heavy food as taken in lunch or dinner in Breakfast. Make it light, small and uncooked natural food items.

By avoiding breads and cooked foods in the breakfast, you can avoid many diseases or will reduce the chances of diseases.

Make your habit or lifestyle to take cooked food only two times in a day. Lunch & dinner are sufficient for our body.

You can take some fresh juice, fruits, nuts, soup, sprouted items or lemon water in the morning breakfast and evening snacks, but not the cooked food-items.

Best items for the breakfast are fresh-juice, sprouted peanuts/green gram (mung)/wheat/chana, seasonal fruits like cucumber, watermelon, apple, papaya, orange, strawberry, water-soaked nuts like almonds/wall-nuts/cashew-nuts/raisins, curds or a cup of fresh-milk, You may select as per your taste and availability.

Always prefer seasonal fruits- because nature always produces such fruits which are suitable to our body in that season. Fresh guava, carrot, orange, watermelon, strawberry, mango, blue berry etc. are best and cheap in seasons. Taking white sesame seeds and raw garlic every morning is also very helpful in preventing diseases like cough, blood thickness and viruses. If you do not feel very hungry till lunch, then may skip breakfast and may take a glass of water with lemon & honey or any fresh juice.

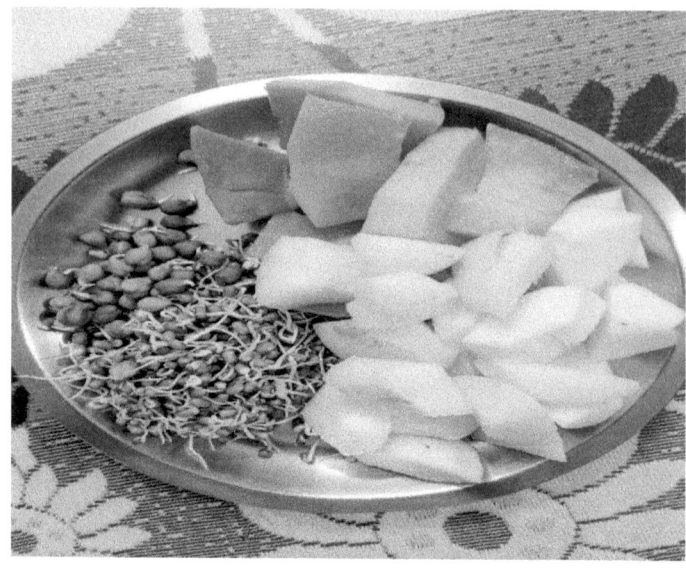

The evening tea & snacks is not very necessary. You may again take fruits or soup, if required. Instead take early dinner. It is advisable that you should go to bed at least two to three hours after the dinner. Because when you sleep the digestion system is very weak. Therefore, for full digestion of your dinner, go to bed at least after two to three hours after dinner.

3. Quality & Quantity of food matters much for being disease-free

3.1. It is the quality of food and the quantity of food we eat, will either make us sick or will protect us from diseases. Healthy food will keep us "healthy" and Junk food will make us "Junk (mean to say sick)"

Please do remember the sayings/proverbs in your life to be disease free:

"We should take food like medicine, otherwise, we will have to take medicine like food"

"We have to take food for living alive, not should live for food"

"If food is good and healthy then why will there be any disease? If food is in oily-spicy-over-cooked-packaged food- fast- junk food/unnatural food, then what medicine will do?"

"In this world, more people die from over-eating than hunger."

"Overeating i.e. eating more than hunger or eating without hunger is the root cause of diseases"

"Eating one bite less is better for good health than to take one bite more than the hunger"

"Diet heals us better than the doctor & medicines"

"There is no medicine like diet. One can be made cured & healthy only by proper regulation of diet."

"During disease we control our food/diet very much. If we control it in our daily routine, why we will get disease."

Better to take food only twice in a day, not eating anything in-between. Set your meal's time as per your daily workload or school/college/office timings.

Always enjoy the food with enough chewing and if possible, take it with family or friends in a pleasant atmosphere.

Never be hurry in taking food, otherwise it will not get proper digested. Give at least 20 to 30 minutes for your lunch or dinner.

The digestion process starts soon after the food enters the mouth, and you are chewing. The salivary glands in our mouth start secreting saliva, which contains enzymes that helps very much in good digestion, hence chew food well.

3.2. The quantity of food you take is also very important. There is only one formula for the quantity of food "you should be feeling hungry at the next time of eating". If you are NOT feeling hungry, DO NOT take any food or may have some juice or lemon-water.

Remember & practice the proverb for your disease-free life "If you have any doubt, whether to take food or not, better not take it and if you feel whether to go to toilet or not, must go"

The quantity of food also depends on the person's age, digestive power, seasons and type of work. Be sure that you take that much food, so that in the next meal, you feel hungry.

3.3. Hunger is the signal of stomach demanding food and for readiness of proper digestion system of your body. As any food is cooked when there is fire, similar is our stomach. Give it food when there is hunger. If you put the pot with raw-food-items for cooking over the stove without lighting the fire, it will never get cooked. Similarly, when you send food in the stomach without hunger, it will not get digested well and will be the cause of many types of diseases.

Thus, have the breakfast in the morning so much that you feel hungry for the lunch in the afternoon. Take that much quantity in the lunch in afternoon so that you feel hungry at dinner time in the evening. There is no need of evening snacks, but better early dinner.

Not eating when we are not hungry, will protect us from many diseases.

4. Take Healthy Food to remain disease free

4.1. The simpler and more natural the food is, the better it is for our body. Natural food means cooked plain food with less oil, ghee and spices having its natural colour preserved even after cooking, more quantity of fruits, salads and sprouted grains/nuts in the meals. (Do not destroy the nutrients in food by cooking too much or frying it too much and adding spices) Avoid non-vegetarian food as much as you can. Vegetarian foods are more natural & suitable to human body, and they protect us more, from many diseases.

Salad has great importance in our daily diet. Take salad or raw onion-cucumber, tomato-carrot etc. in sufficient quantity with food. Sprouted gram or sprouted green gram is very good for our health in addition to the salad.

Always take some rest after lunch at noon and walk after dinner in the night. "After lunch rest a while, after dinner walk a mile" is the proverb useful for our daily life- adopt it & make it a routine of your daily-life.

Wash your hands properly before eating. Also, urinating after meals reduces the chances of urinary tract diseases.

4.2. Eat live/healthy food

There is a saying that if you plant an apple tree then how you can expect oranges from it, in fact what you will sow seeds accordingly you will reap.

I mean to say that you can never hope to remain healthy & disease-free by eating lifeless, packaged, stale, much oily & fried, fried-dead, junk food, it will definitely make you sick.

By dead food I mean food whose elements have been destroyed in the process of preparation or cooking or which are cooked long before and packed for sell, things fried in oil, vitamins and minerals roasted in fire with a lot of chillies and spices, old vegetables, polished and dusted white Rice, bran removed flour, white sugar, stale rice and baker's bread, old withered vegetables, ready to eat packed vegetables, etc. Junk food and fast food like noodles pizza burger etc. are also not healthy food and they lead to obesity and many diseases even if they feel good to eat for some time.

To be healthy and disease free, eat vital/live food. Vital foods are bread made from flour with bran in own kitchen, rice with red particles, steamed carrot, beans & peas, milk, green vegetables, fresh seasonal fruits, sprouted gram-wheat-peanuts, honey, cucumber, tomato onion salad etc..

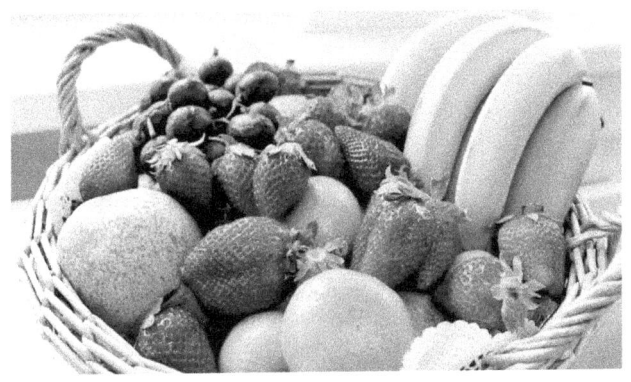

Be sure to take a handful of sprouted gram/green moong/ peanuts or wheat every day in breakfast or lunch because it is the most vital, live food, it also contains vitamin E in abundance

By regular consumption of live or vital fresh & hot cooked healthy homemade food, fruits, vegetables, juices, salad etc. we can be safe from diseases or will be healed by taking proper such foods advised by a dietician or naturopathy doctor.

4.3. How should our food be? In this regard, medical experts advise to eat such food which are: -

(a) Fresh and easily digestible.

(b) Should be non-irritating to the mouth & stomach - that is, which does not cause burning sensation, cramps or excitement in the stomach, like very chilli-spicy vegetables, very sour curd, etc.

(c) Should be a mild laxative & fibrous, the food with enough fibre, does not get stuck in the stomach or intestines, does not cause constipation.

(d) Which purifies the blood (body), i.e. it is alkaline. Any disease occurs due to increase in the proportion of acidity in the blood. To be healthy and disease free, we have to take 4 parts of alkali-rich and one part of acid-rich food in our daily diet.

Acid producing food is - all types of meat, sweets, sugar, tea, jam-jelly, too-much-white-salt, most of the packaged food & juice, tobacco, soda water, cold drinks, food fried in oil and ghee, intoxicating drinks, chocolate etc.

Alkali producing food is- green leafy vegetables, fruits, radish, carrot, spinach, onion, turnip, grapes, fig, pear, lemon, cucumber, tomato, amla, ripe banana, strawberry, dates, melon, beetroot, bottle-gourd, bitter gourd, green fresh peas, leafy-vegetables, broccoli, and sprouted grains etc.

Therefore, include more green vegetables, salad, seasonal fruits, sprouted grains, jaggery or honey, milk in your diet and avoid dead-food like white polished rice & flour, sugar & sugar product, meat, stale food, junk food etc. If there is enough of alkaline items in the food, we will remain far away from diseases.

(e) Nutritious food whose nutrients have not been destroyed during the process of preparation or cooking. Therefore, take fresh food in natural condition as much as possible.

But keep one thing in mind that if even nutritious food is taken without hunger, not digested in the stomach properly, your body does not assimilate it and convert it into blood, then it is also useless for you. Therefore, through practice and experience, decide on nutritious food suitable for your body.

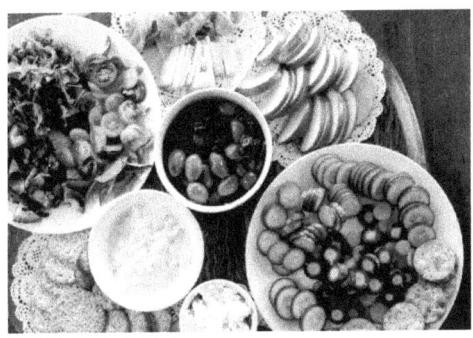

(f) The food must be enjoyable to eat to you. Or develop interest in that food. feel pleasure in eating the food Which helps in digestion. The pleasure or happiness in eating that food is directly related to our mind, and the mind is related to the fluids of the digestive system. When we eat with a happy mind, digestive fluids are secreted in sufficient quantity. On the contrary, unpleasant food causes irritability. The release of digestive fluids and internal secretions of the body is linked to eating in a pleasant mood and enjoying the food.

Taking food in anxiety, worry, sadness, fear, hurry, under-pressure etc. affects directly on our digestive system. In this situation, instead of benefit from food, it harms our body.

(g) Change food items in your daily diet as much as it is possible. By this, all types of nutrients and vitamins will also be available. Eating the same type of food daily without change leads to monotony and interest starts to wane. Therefore, If you eat bread daily, then have rice once a week. Sometimes breakfast consists of cereals then sometimes fruits. Today the bread is made of wheat, tomorrow it is made of corn. Change the vegetables every day.

Avoid dishes like pizza-noodles-burgers-cold drinks-French fry potato, because these are acidic (causing diseases) and cause great harm to the stomach.

4.4. Ways to prepare food and clean kitchen

It is the practical experience of doctors that your kitchen is also a medical clinic. Those whose kitchens are smelly, utensils are dirty, knives and utensils are dirty, cobwebs/insects and dirt are found in flour, rice and spices, then definitely disease will come in that home. If you want to remain healthy then first keep kitchen & food items clean, it does not cost any money.

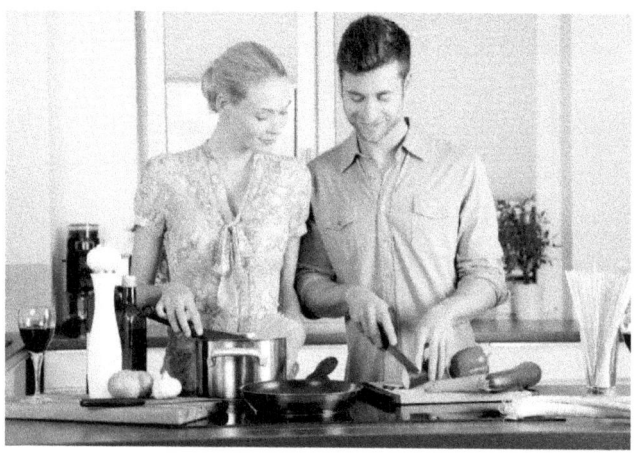

The health also depends on the way food is prepared. Such as washing vegetables thoroughly before cutting them (washing after cutting is a bad habit), do not peel vegetables & fruits unnecessarily, do not mash them with rice, do not make vegetables juicy, do not destroy nutrients by frying vegetables. Cook any ingredient by covering it. Be sure to serve radish-amla-mint-coriander chutney and some salad like onion-tomato-cabbage-spinach-coriander-radish etc. with the food. Eat food hot and in small portions. Keep food, milk, water etc. covered and do not allow flies & insects, oil slickers, spiders or lizards to sit on them.

Pay full attention to the cleanliness of the cloth, dishes, knives used in the kitchen.

Cooking food in pressure cooker is good from health point of view. In its absence, use lidded utensils and low flame.

4.5. Bring changes in food according to season, age & person

Honey and potatoes are not so good in summer, milk in rainy season, whereas in winter they are beneficial. Digestion process is slow in rainy season and fast in winter. In summer, more liquids and juicy fruits are required, while in winter, heavy food like nuts, milk, jaggery is required. Therefore, change the diet according to the season.

The form of food according to the person i.e. the condition of the person will change. The quantity and type of food for children, youth and old people will be different. Differentiate the food according to the person's body also. If the stomach is constipated, then laxative, puffed rice, crunchy foods will be suitable, vegetables with their peels will be prepared, roti should be made by mixing bran. If there is dysentery in the stomach, then wetting and astringent substances like curd, bel, ripe banana etc. If there is a gas disorder then dry food should be taken, if there is phlegm then anti-phlegm like bread, vegetables should be taken, if there is bile then one should take sour fruits like orange etc. For one person, honey or jaggery in curd would be appropriate, for another person salt and cumin. Therefore, decide according to the person, age, time and season. Also keep in mind what to take in the morning and what to take in the evening. Generally, sprouted grains is good in the morning & daytime, harmful at night. In this regard, consult a naturopath or dietician for advice or read a diet-related book or decide on your own diet suitable for your body through practice and experience.

5.NOT Eating in-between (Don't Make Stomach a Dustbin)

Please do not eat anything between two meals. If a train is running or standing on one line/track and another train is sent on it, then an accident is certain, and both the trains will be damaged. Similarly, if there is one food in your stomach under digestion and you send another in it, then it is certain that you will get diseases.

<u>Do not make the stomach a dustbin- sending food and drinks whenever you like or get. Give time to your stomach to get digested the food earlier sent by you</u>

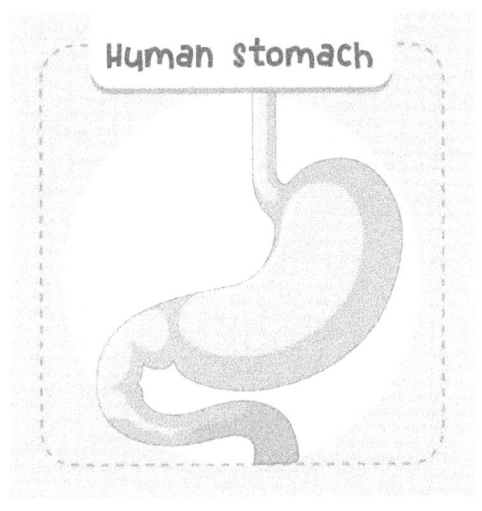

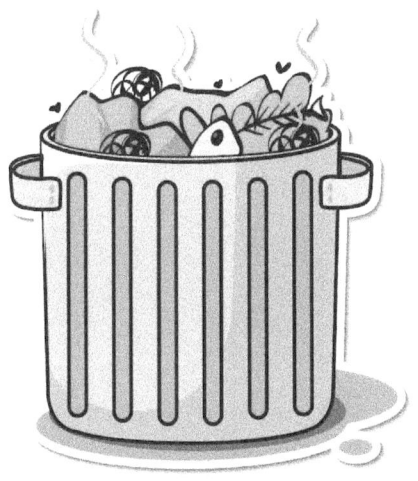

After you eat, it takes about six to eight hours for food to pass through your stomach and small intestine. Food then enters your large intestine (colon) for further digestion, absorption of water and, finally, elimination of undigested food. It takes about 36 hours for food to move through the entire colon.

Therefore, if you wish to never have any disease, please do not eat in between two meals. Keep a gap of at least 6 hours between two meals. It should be our habit that we should eat only when we feel hungry and at fixed time in a day- maximum two meals and one light breakfast. Never eat more than your hunger. <u>A little bit less eating than the hunger is better than overeating.</u>

Take lunch and dinner at a fixed time every day. This will release the juice/enzyme from your stomach to digest food so that whatever you eat will be digested properly and you will remain healthy. If for some reason you cannot take food at that particular time, then take some soup, fruit juice or fruit, but do not take any food between two meals.

Sometimes, on special occasions, one has to eat heavy food or many types of dishes, in such a situation it is certain that one does not feel hungry at the time of the second meal, then remember the formula "If there is doubt Eat or not eat, it is better not to eat".

6.Drink Enough water- Fresh and Potable

Water is body's main chemical component and makes up about 50% to 70% of our body weight. Our body depends on water to survive. Water not only required for maintenance of our body system, but it also helps taking out the toxins out of our body in different forms (urine or sweat) to keep us disease free.

Every cell, tissue, blood and organ in our body needs water to work properly. Water is necessary for getting rid of wastes through urination/sweating/bowel movements, keeping our temperature normal, lubricating and cushions joints, protecting sensitive tissues and keeping us hydrated.

Lack of water can lead to dehydration. Even mild dehydration can drain our energy and make you tired.

Therefore, it is very necessary to use safe, clean and potable drinking & cooking water for us and also clean water for bathing to be disease-free.

Contaminants in our water can lead to many health issues, including jaundice, diarrhoea, other liver & stomach problems, gastrointestinal illness, reproductive problems, and neurological disorders. Infants, young children, pregnant women, the elderly, and people with weakened immune systems may be at increased risk for becoming sick after drinking contaminated water. For example, elevated levels of arsenic, lead, dusts, chemicals can cause serious health problems.

Hence be assured that our household and workplace drinking water is clean and potable. Better to take water from government supply, deep-hand pumps and deep borings. Get our household water tested through Public Health & Engineering Department or whichever source is possible and feasible for you.

You can also judge the water purity to some extent by its taste, colour, sedimentation if there is any after keeping water for some time and smell. But its chemical & other tests are necessary to be in the safer side about its purity and potability from reasonable sources & methods. Different types of filters and water-purifiers are also available in the market for making our drinking & cooking water safe and hygienic. In some conditions using boiled water for drinking is one of the solution.

Taking bath in clean water is also very necessary to be safe from skin diseases.

Quantity of water for our body in daily life

Every day we lose water through our breath, sweat, urine and bowel movements. For our body to function properly, we must replenish its water supply by drinking water, juice, milk, beverages and foods & fruits that contain water. About 20% of daily fluid intake usually comes from food and the rest from drinks.

There is different opinion for quantity of water we should take daily. It depends upon season, place/environment, type of work, for women if they are feeding child, and age. But in general, we should drink 2 to 3 litters of water daily besides food, juice, fruits like watermelon or berries, milk, tea or coffee, other drinks etc. Minimum 8 glasses of water are recommended by most of dietitians to take daily.

In case of diseases like diarrhoea, loose-motion, vomiting, dehydration large quantity of water is required to our body, for which strictly follow the instructions of your doctor or health-professional.

The quantity of water is enough or not can be also judged in general by colour of our urine which should be colourless like water or very light yellow, thirst you feel and whether you are going for urination after every 3 to 4 hours during daytime.

When to drink water and about food & eating habits

It is my experience that do not drink water between meals, nor eat too juicy/liquid/gravy/watery food. Juicy food cannot be chewed sufficiently. Due to being like liquid, it immediately goes down the throat into stomach due to which the digestive saliva of the mouth does not get mixed as desired and hence the food is not digested properly. Due to poor digestion in the stomach, it becomes heavy and gassy. Remember digestion process starts from mouth, and if a food is more time in the mouth in the process of proper & sufficient chewing, it gets more digestive.

A person who wishes to remain healthy forever should separate water and food. I mean to say take food or cook food as much as it can be dry (not much gravy/watery), keep the vegetable or dish as dry as possible – do not make it too juicy.

Chew bread or rice or main food thoroughly and then eat pulses or vegetables separately. In this way, adequate amount of digestive saliva will be mixed in the food, and it will be digested properly.

Drink water one hour before or one hour after meals. Try to take as less water during eating meals as you can, but drinking enough water in a day is very important for the body and to remain healthy.

Be sure to drink potable safe fresh water throughout the day. Two glasses of warm water in the morning before defecation, one glass of water one hour after breakfast, one glass one hour before lunch, one glass one hour after lunch, one glass in the evening, two-three times before dinner. Drink water after and before sleeping.

Drink water at your body temperature:

Always take water at your body temperature or little warm as much as possible. The very cold water from the refrigerator may feel good but ultimately it is harmful. Similarly cold-drinks or juice with ice is harmful for the health. Therefore, you should make a practice of drinking plain or fresh water of your body temperature. Give up cold drinks and replace them with fruit juice or buttermilk or lemon water or fresh coconut water.

7. Have Fresh & clean Air to be disease free

Air, Water and Food are the 3 major essential intakes to keep our body fit and healthy. If these all are clean, fresh, healthy, enough, then you will be certainly disease free.

In paragraphs above, you have gone through the instructions on food and water, please take precaution for the air too which you breath.

Kindly refer the key facts mentioned in the World Health Organization website (https://www.who.int/news-room/fact-sheets/detail/ambient-(outdoor)-air-quality-and-health#:~:text=Air%20pollution%20is%20one%20of,acute%20respiratory%20diseases%2C%20including%20asthma.)

- Air pollution is one of the greatest environmental risk to health. By reducing air pollution levels, countries can reduce the burden of disease from stroke, heart disease, lung cancer, and both chronic and acute respiratory diseases, including asthma.
- The combined effects of ambient air pollution and household air pollution are associated with 6.7 million premature deaths annually.
- Ambient (outdoor) air pollution is estimated to have caused 4.2 million premature deaths worldwide in 2019.

Therefore, it is very necessary for us to be disease free that we breath fresh & clean air, in our home, at workplace and out-door too. Always keep away from place where there is air-pollution. Use masks or other tools where there is any air-pollution to have a safe breathing. Make your home with enough windows and ventilators, similar be your workplace/study centres. Sleep in a room with enough ventilation of fresh air.

Your kitchen should be also well ventilated that no smoke remains inside to be inhaled.

Do not burn mosquito-sticks or other repellent in your sleeping room in the night but better to use mosquito-net. Similarly, do not burn fire or use room-heater during winter inside the sleeping room with door closed. They generate carbon-dioxide absorbing oxygen, and more quantity of CO_2 in the room may kill us.

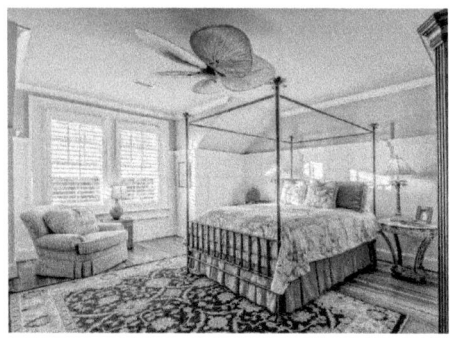

Plant trees and flowers in your home garden to give you clean air with enough oxygen.

Have a walk in the evening or morning in the lawn where there is fresh air, not by the side of roads where many vehicles are running at that time.

8. Understand the Safety Signals of your Body and let them clean your body

We take cold, cough, fever, headache, vomiting, diarrhoea, boils and pimples etc. as a disease but they are actually the safety signals of accumulation of toxins inside our body. Instead of suppressing them, let the toxins of our body come out and clean our body. Instead of treating them as your enemy, take them as a friend and strength of your body's immune system.

Understand that they are nature's notice to you of the accumulated toxins in your body, and, of future acute diseases if not taken precaution. They are also the natural process of purifying our body throwing out toxic elements accumulated inside us as per our immune system.

The biggest wonder of nature is our body which has thousands of veins, arteries, bones, which are amazingly connected to each other. The heartbeat that starts at birth continues to beat like an automatic machine until death. Sense organs like eyes and skin experience happiness and sorrow. Along with these, nature has made adequate immunity arrangements/system in our body to keep us healthy.

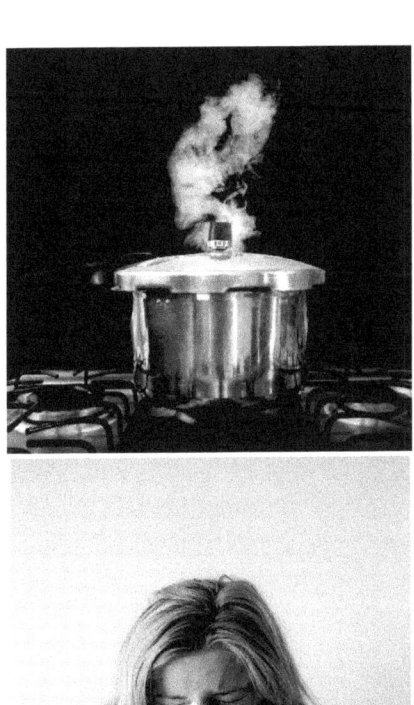

One form of our body's disease-protective-system is cold, cough, body-pain, headache, dysentery, fever, boils etc. When more foreign matter (toxic elements) accumulates in our body, it gets expelled in the form of phlegm, mucus, faeces, sweat, urine, pus, causing fever, cold, cough, headache, wounds, diarrhoea etc. If you do not disturb these nature's process of purifying your body, you will never suffer from chronic and fatal diseases.

Hence you should welcome those signals of accumulation of toxic elements in our body and try to purify your body instead of suppressing them by medicines. In case/time of these immune signals, you should take adequate rest, skip one or two meals, take soup & fresh-juice, hot lemon-water, avoid un-healthy foods & drinks, and allow your body to throw out accumulated toxic elements. After this you will feel fresh & energized.

<u>Just as when too much pressure builds up in a pressure cooker, the safety valve bursts and the pressure is released, similarly the above signals which we think as diseases are the safety valves of the body and are the means to remove the disorders & toxins accumulated in the body.</u>

To remain healthy forever, fasting for once a month giving rest to your stomach or skipping a meal replacing taking only fruits & vegetables-soup for one time a week is beneficial for the body. Like machines, the digestive system also needs a day or an evening's rest, so that it can do its work properly. If complete fasting is not possible, you can spend your day on honey water or seasonal fruit juice or vegetable soup and have some fruits in the evening. But one should not fast if has diseases like blood pressure, anaemia, tuberculosis, cancer etc. Instead of that you can eat fruits/juices taking suggestions from the doctor.

<u>Great physicians say that acute disease (toxic-accumulation-signals) is a friend, not an enemy.</u> There are several examples around us that suppressing such body-purifying light disease, we get chronic disease or over-medication for suppression of such signals, causes too much harm to our lever-kidney-lungs.

There is no harm in taking medicine or going to hospital or consulting doctors you trust, to save life in an emergency, but after that the body should be purified by good healthy diets and other actions mentioned in the paragraphs above.

Instead of allopathic chemical medicines, I would suggest, based on my long experiences, that first give preference to naturopathy or homeopathy healing system. In them there are least quantity of medicines or herbs going inside our body. Acupressure, physiotherapy and yoga-asanas are another healing system with no medicines but is not suitable for all types of health-problems. But wherever suitable give preference to these. Then my suggestion will be for ayurvedic-Unani-Chinese-home-remedies treatments because they have minimum side effects. Always avoid painkillers-medicines easily available in the market with lots of luring advertisements, which are very harmful for our lever, kidney and stomach. In case of emergency, use them as minimum as you can.

9. Quit/Control Sugar, Tea, Smoking & Alcohol

Sugar is like a "white poison" (means to say very harmful for our body) is suggestion of many doctors, heath-professionals and naturopaths. It is my own experience too that Sugar is very harmful for our body and is also the root cause of many diseases. Therefore, if you want to remain healthy and disease free, then you must give up sugar completely or take it in very controlled quantity.

Use jaggery and honey instead of sugar. Jaggery and honey contain natural properties and essential elements for our body. Avoid sweets etc. made of sugar as far as possible or consume them in very controlled quantities. Whenever you take it in small quantity, make sure to take cloves and cardamom along with it. Clove cardamom will reduce the toxicity of sugar in sweets to some extent.

If you want to never fall sick, then give up tea, coffee, cigarette, alcohol, wine, drugs and tobacco along with sugar. Tea, coffee, cigarette, alcohol, wine and tobacco all harm our body and cause diseases including cancer. Then why should you take these? Do not take such dangerous items to health for a status symbol. If you are taking them in party or meetings, then take them in a very controlled quantity with enough healthy diets to compensate the harm caused by them to our body.

Instead of tea & coffee, you can take many types of fresh juices, coconut-water or soup. Instead of tea & coffee, you can give lemon water, juice, fruits, nuts, etc to the guests to welcome them.

If you want to drink something during work time or in the morning and evening, then you can take soup or coconut-water or fruit juice or curd-water, hot milk etc. Mix hot milk with turmeric powder-pinch of black-pepper powder and take it with honey or jaggery at night. There are many

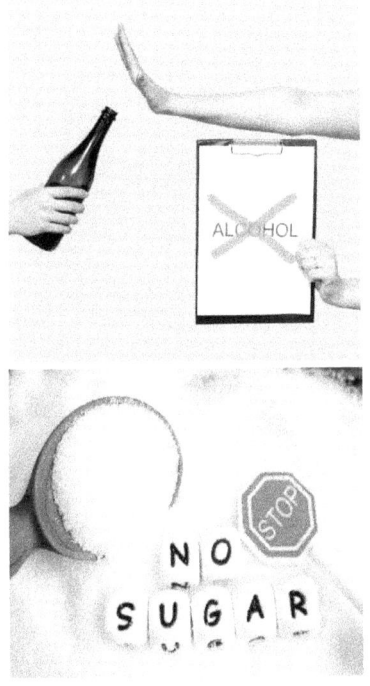

advertisements about healthy energy drinks in TV & Newspapers but be careful to them. Most of them contains sugar, added salt, preservatives etc. and are harmful. Golden-milk (milk with turmeric powder with a pinch of black-pepper powder) is very good for health, improving our immune system as well as giving us energy.

50 percent of chances of getting disease can be reduced only by giving up sugar, wine/alcohol, tea-coffee, cigarettes, tobacco, drugs etc.. This is an experiment conducted on thousands of patients, not just a sermon.

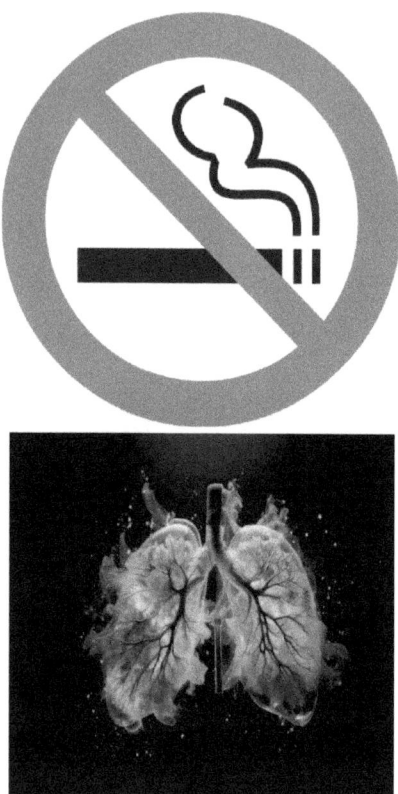

You will find many examples of this in your daily life: heavy cigarette smokers are suffering from heart and lung diseases and alcoholics are suffering from liver problems. Much Tea & coffee drinkers from drowsiness, lack of sleep, gastric. Tobacco chewer suffering from mouth cancer. The first thing any doctor says is to leave them. You should also give up these completely to remain healthy and fit always. Do not fall prey to the lure of false civilization, advertisements and personality-show off. Most of the people use wine and cigarettes to show their nobility, richness or to hide their inferiority complex, which becomes life-threatening for them. Develop habits that help prevent diseases and bring sustainable happiness to you.

10. Avoid Accidents, Infections, Disability and Strokes

Significant percentage of the people who come to the hospital, to doctor and spend money on medicines, are victims of some accidents or suffer from some disability. If you want, you can avoid up to 90% of accidents and disability, just by taking necessary precautions.

Rushing down the stairs, turning around suddenly, having moss in the bathroom, spilling water or oil on the floor and walking hastily at such a places, many a times become the cause of fractures and accidents – which you can avoid by taking required precautions.

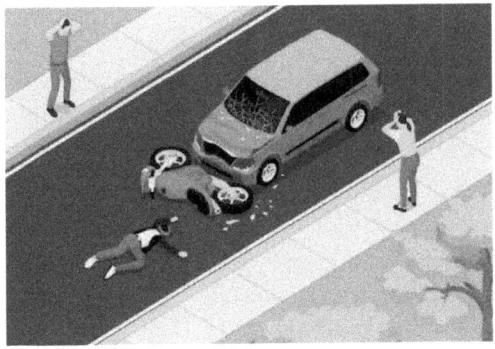

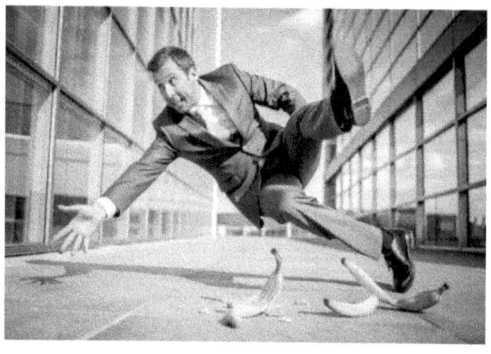

Following the traffic rules you can avoid accidents on roads. Driving at high speed, driving after taking wine, driving while listening to loud music or using mobile phone while driving, not using helmets while driving motorcycle are the causes of most of the accidents due to which we lose our limbs or get head-injury, become victims of untimely death. Be late than never. Also, due to our hurry to reach fast, not starting to destination taking enough time, driving in the night & getting sudden sleep, or our carelessness driving, most of the accidents happen and we reach the hospital and death's door.

Similarly, during pregnancy, not taking pre-natal & post-natal vaccination & care, not eating proper food, not avoiding diseases & excess weight at time of pregnancy, lifting heavy weights, not visiting doctors regularly, not having delivery at hospital/nursing homes under supervision of qualified doctors can cause disability or malnutrition or untimely death of the child. By following the precautions suggested by health workers and doctors before, during and after delivery, we can keep ourselves and our future child and mother healthy and free from disability. Marriages in very close relation, also causes child's disability. The disability of the child/any person is mostly due to our mistake & carelessness – which we can prevent.

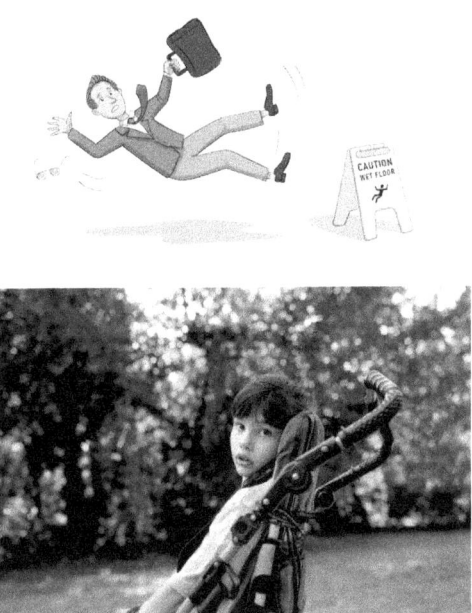

We can protect ourselves from Corona and such other viruses & infections by becoming careful, keeping physical distance, using of mask, washing hands with soap from time to time, cleaning hands with sanitizer after touching or taking bath and by increasing the immunity of our body, we can be saved.

In old age, due to ageing, hearing loss, joint pains, vision-loss, cataract etc. is very common. But we can minimise the effects and diseases coming in old age by healthy habits while young mentioned above and using proper aids & appliances.

11. Importance of Rest & stress-free life to be disease-free

Literally the meaning of Disease is Dis-ease i.e. "lack of ease". Rest is as important as food for our body's good health. The main cause of many diseases is lack of rest. In fact, lack of adequate rest and sleep causes many types of diseases.

Four types of rest are necessary (a) After meals some rest for few minutes or during work a short break (b) Sleeping at night after a long day's work (c) Weekend holidays in schools & offices and (d) going on site-seeing tour or meeting other family members in other parts of the country in a year after many month of works or study.

At least 7 to 8 hours of sleep, depending on age and type of work, is compulsory for our body to remain healthy & disease-free. If you work on a computer, give rest to your eyes for at least 5 minutes after every two hours. Decide working hours according to your age. If you have to work sitting, then take a walk for ten minutes after every two hours. Even if you are studying, take some rest after an hour or two. Go and take a glass of fresh water at your body temperature.

In the absence of adequate rest, there is extra burden on the body and mind, the consequences of which are that we fall sick, life expectancy decreases, our nature becomes irritable, and many diseases related to mind, stomach, liver, kidney and brain occurs.

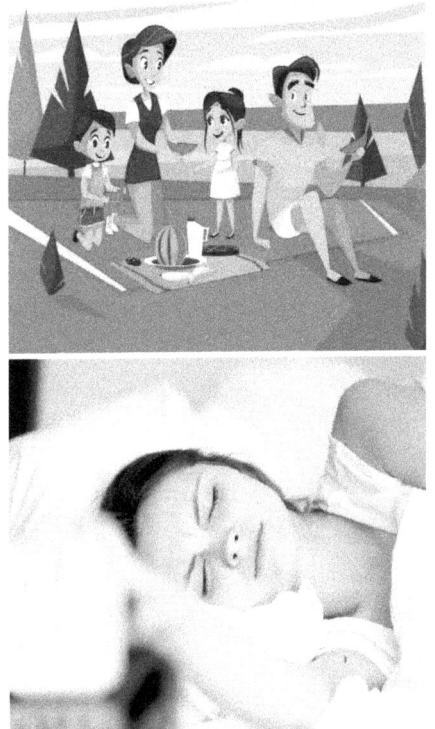

Enjoy some entertainment after work in the evening. Go to park on a walk or on drive with spouse & children in the evening. Have some physical exercise. Watch favourite TV-show or listen to music, play with friends, or read some magazine of your interest. It will also give us new strength and energy to work the next day.

For uninterrupted sleep, before sleeping, wash your hands and feet with hot water (in summers, wash them with cold water), urinate and leave aside all the worries and sleep on a hard mattress, keeping your spine straight. The sleeping room should be airy and clean. Sleeping early and waking up early is good for health. One should sleep at least two hour after the dinner. Make sure to use mosquito net while sleeping. Mosquitoes are the cause of many diseases like malaria, dengue etc. Do not use mosquito-coils or liquid, which gas we inhale while sleeping which are dangerous for health and lungs.

In 12 months of the year, take out at least one week or ten days (as suitably available to you), to go for tour and site-seeing with your family/children/friends, taking leave from the work or during you vacations in school/college/institution. It will give you a new energy and peace of mind for continuing your job/study with more stamina & energy. It is also necessary for your good health and well-being.

Have a Stress-free life & helping attitude

One of the main causes of diseases like insomnia or sleeplessness, mental diseases and many other troubles like depression/anxiety/stress, generally comes due to worry, competition, jealousy and unnatural life. If you get upset after seeing other's house or salary or clothes or car, if you get jealous seeing relative's or friend's property or success, then your body & mind will get stressed and you will fall sick, there will be no harm to them.

Many times, mishappening to own family members like accident or heart-attack or death or such sad-news causes shock and mental tension. Also, failure in exam or in love-affairs or in business or in stock-market causes such stress to mind. But if you can trust "God", as suggested to do in the morning prayer (mentioned in the step 1 in the beginning of this chapter), believe it that it was God's wish. For any incidence, which is not in our control, accept it as God's wish and console your mind, do not let tension & stress to overcome you. Win such stress, tension & sadness by strength of your willpower and mind. If it was not in your control, by being in stress & tension, what you will do??? By getting in tension or mentally disturbed, you will harm yourselves and your other family members. Think over it and be calm in such cases. Take steps to fulfil the gap and solve the consequences arise due to sad incidence you had not expected.

The practice of forgiving and forgetting (Forget and Forgive) will eliminate your mental stress and the number of friends will start increasing. Always have a helping attitude, which sometimes you may also need.

This does not mean that you should stop working hard, improving the standard of living and opposing injustice. But do it with a calm and simple mind, without any tension, jealousy, worry or hatred. Then it will not have any bad effect on your health.

By having faith in God or on your respectful person, accepting whatever happens as God's wish and judgement, we can avoid stress, and the diseases caused by stress & sadness. If something miss-happen to me, I believe that it is the God's wish and will be good for me. In Hindi, it is famous song "Ye mat socho kal kya hoga, jo bhi hoga achcha hoga" means "Do not bother what will happen tomorrow- whatever will happen it will be good for me". Practicing it in my life, I have found a great peace of mind and can remain stress-free. Practice it and you too will find peace of mind leading to good health.

Again, I want to repeat that do not bother or be sad for the incidence, which is not in your jurisdiction or control. Ignoring such incidence will give you peace of mind and save you from unnecessary stress.

Also, keep away from infections. We have to take necessary precautions against infectious/transmittable diseases and with our wisdom, we can stay safe from them.

Keep one more thing in mind that sorrow decreases by sharing and happiness increases by sharing. If you are feeling sad, share it with your trusted family members, friends or teacher. If you are a parent, a teacher, someone's friend, then take care of your children, students and friends and support them in their grief or stress, lighten their sorrow, console them and help them to overcome grief and stress. They will also help you in your need.

Make a habit to visit if someone of your friend or relative is sick or in trouble or in pain. Go with a flower or fruits or a relevant greeting card if suitable for that occasion. It gives a great relief and strength to sick person or a person in pain or trouble than medicines. Never forget to thanks for any help you get. Never hesitate to ask excuse if you have hurt someone or done any mistake. Never forget to wish someone you know on their birthday/ marriage/ anniversary etc. Such good habits make number of friends in need and save us from mental stress and disease.

12. Be Optimistic and Give some time for social cause & philanthropic initiatives

We have come in this earth empty handed and will depart empty handed. We all are mortal and leaving this world one day. We will be remembered only by our good work & behaviour, helping attitudes, kindness, due to our philanthropic works and devoting time & contribution to social cause. As mentioned earlier the sorrow halves by sharing while happiness doubles by sharing. Social works and philanthropic initiatives give us Happiness, and Satisfaction which are also helpful for our good health, peace of mind and a meaningful life.

Human being is a social-animal, and we take a lot from the society, hence it is our duty to give something back to the society. The joy and happiness you will experience in Giving & Sharing, will also keep you happy and healthy.

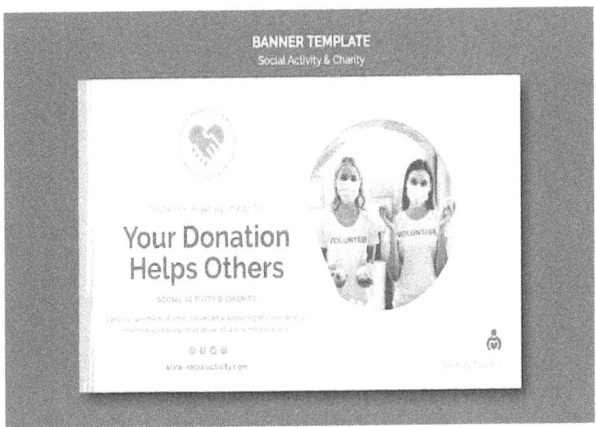

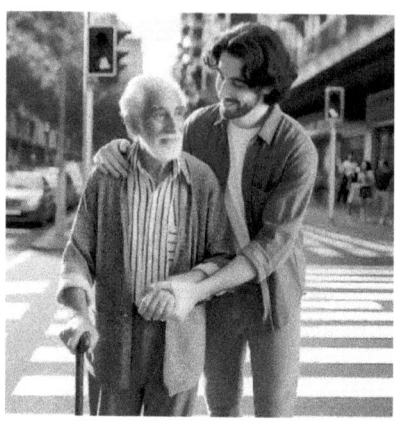

Do whatever you can to help your neighbours, friends, people and those in distress. At least you can console them. At least you can visit them when they are sick or in trouble. You can help a blind person or small children to cross the road. You can help an old person for bringing his/her grocery or medicines if required. You may be also helped in your troubles (which will happen to you at some point or the other), which you will need at that time.

Never forget to express gratitude and thanks to someone who helps or serves you.

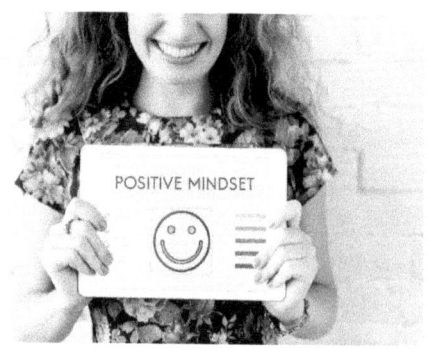

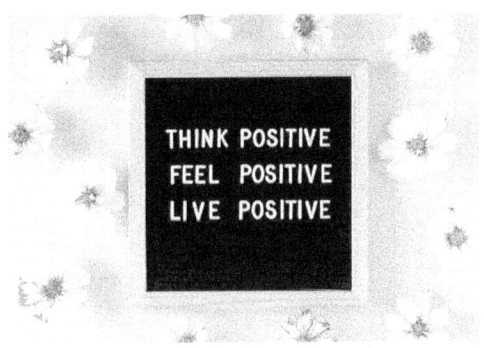

An optimistic & positive nature will keep you happy and healthy. You will get more friends and supporters. While becoming pessimistic and having negative attitude will harm you, not others. You will lose friends and relatives criticizing them and having a fault-finding attitude. As you enter the home through the doors while walls are there in much more space than door. Similarly see the good qualities of a person, to enter him meaning to win him as your friend, ignoring his/her weaknesses & bad habits. You do good to everyone; it will make you satisfied and your life meaningful.

But remember one thing, 'do good and put it in the river', I mean to say, do charity not with the feeling of "reward", do it only with the feeling of "benevolence", because only detached charity is pleasant and enjoyable.

Nav Bharat Jagriti Kendra is a well-known most credible voluntary organization working since last 53 years in India for poor, destitute, marginalized community, person in distress & mental illness, girls' education, eradication of avoidable blindness etc. I am one of its founder member. You can connect with its social philanthropic programs & works through the website www.nbjk.org or email satishgirija@nbjk.org. Get more information by contacting +919431140508. You may also get connected with other charities as suitable for you. Spare some time and share something for the poor & marginalized community and experience the "joy of giving" yourselves. The peace of mind, satisfaction and happiness are very important to us to remain disease free.

Again, to recapture the points for attention

1.Change a little your Morning Routine ((Blessings, Warm water, Ganesh Kriya, Splashing and Yoga)

2.The Break-fast (No Cooked Food in Breakfast)

3. Quality & Quantity of food matters much

4. Take Healthy Food to remain disease free

5.NO Eating in-between (Don't Make Stomach a Dustbin)

6.Drink Enough water- Fresh and Potable

7. Have Fresh & clean Air to be disease free

8. Understand the Safety Signals of your Body and let them clean your body

9. Quit/Control Sugar, Tea, Smoking & Alcohol

10. Avoid Accidents, Infections, Disability and Strokes

11. Importance of Rest & stress-free life to be disease-free

12. Be Optimistic and Give some time for social cause & philanthropic initiatives

CHAPTER 2

Time management & A Sample Daily Routine/timetable to living Disease free

(You make your own daily routine/timetable as suitable to your work and follow it strictly. It is wise to plan your day for a better use of the time)

Time management and discipline in own's life is very necessary to be free from any diseases and have a happy life. Here I am giving a sample, but you shall have your own as per your age, profession and suitability.

6.00 AM: Getting up after a 7 to 8 hours sleep

6.00 AM to 6.03 AM: Prayer on your bed with closed eyes with joint hands upon your chest for blessings remembering God whom you worship. Pray for a meaningful and happy day in your own way or saying "You" are almighty, and "You" know what is good for me. I trust "you", whatever will be in the day, it will be good for me. Help me to get my work done perfectly with full honesty and sincerity. Let me be kind and merciful to others, as "You" are to me. Help me so that I achieve my target and ambition……..Aameen"

6.03- 6.10 AM: Say good morning to others whom you see with a smile.

Drink two to three glasses of warm water. May squeeze a lemon in it with pinch of rock-salt and black-pepper powder. Then walk in the room/balcony/on lawn-grass of your house with foot without sleepers/bare-foot for 5 -10 minutes. Hope you will get pressure for the toilet.

6.10 to 6.25: Toilet and then Ganesh Kriya & Ashwini Mudra then bath. (You follow the process of Ganesh Kriya and Ashwini Mudra, as explained in this book or see it doing in YouTube or read it how performed searching on google with its benefits). For this you have to make an arrangement of water in the toilet for soaking your left-hand middle finger in water for Ganesh-kriya & washing your hands cleaning inner-anus, and after defecation, instead of using tissue-paper.

Then brush your teeth with good paste. Splash cold clean water on your open eyes with mouth full of water after brush.

Then take bath. During bath, first put normal water on your lower part of the stomach for 1 minute rubbing with your palms clockwise. Then take water on backside & middle of your head for 1 minute. Then on whole body. Never put hot water on head & eyes. Try to use cold water in summer and Luke-warm in winter for bathing.

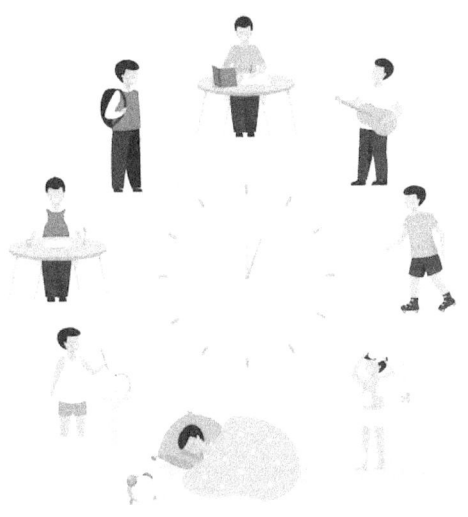

6.25 to 6.55: Yoga/ Asan/ jogging/ walking/playing outdoor game like badminton or tennis on open fresh air where there is no pollution.

6.55 to 8.00: Reading good books of great person or self - study for one hour for your better career

8.00 to 8.20: Breakfast. Take night-soaked two full wallnuts & 4 pieces of almonds with 2-3 pieces of garlic-cloves. Then take handful of sprouted green-gram or hoarse-gram with sprouted peanuts. Eat one apple having thin skin cutting it with teeth (not by knife), some ripen papaya, banana and some strawberry, guava, watermelon, cucumber or such seasonal fruits. Then fresh juice of orange or milkshake or curd or hot-milk with honey and a pinch of turmeric & pepper-powder in the hot milk.

8.20: Departure for workplace or school-college

(Go to workplace/school/college on foot if close by or by bi-cycle or otherwise by public-transport if is convenient. Less-use private car to save pollution of the environment.

9.30 AM to 5.00 PM Woking/ studying. Take – 2-3 glasses of water at body-temperature during work or study. Rest your eyes at every 2 hours if working over computer for 5-10 minutes. Walk a little at every 2 hours if your job is of sitting type.

Lunch in-between 12.30 PM to 1.30 PM. In Lunch have home-cooked breads, dry-vegetables without many spices, enough salads of onion-cucumber-tomato-carrot-green salad-leaves etc. with sprouted chana or moong (green-gram). Drink minimum water during lunch. Better take water 30 minutes before lunch and 30 minutes after lunch.

5.30 PM to 7.30 PM: Reaching home. Have some fresh juice of seasonal fruits or coconut water. Recreation by walking on park with children & family, playing games with friends & family, dancing, playing musical-instruments, swimming if swimming pool available, jogging, visiting friends or any out-door activity as suitable etc.

7.30-8.00 PM: Dinner with family. Have again home-cooked hot food, enough salads. Water 30 minutes before or after. Milk or curd or fresh juice.

8.00 PM to 10.00 PM: Self -study, Watching TV. Or other essential work at home.

10.00 PM: Brush your teeth. Wash your feet with warm water or if suitable have a bath with Luke-warm water. Have a glass of hot milk with turmeric powder. Remember your God you worship thanking for a meaningful day. Then go to bed in a room having good ventilation of clean fresh air. Have mosquito net on bed instead of burning coils if there are mosquitos in the room. Use ortho-hard-mattress on bed for sleeping.

*Drink at least 3 litres of water in a day. Avoid wines and smoking. Throw-out sugar from the home/kitchen and replace it with jaggery (Gud) and pure honey. Use rock-salt instead of white-salt. Have kitchen very clean. All food-items & drinking water covered.

Rinse your mouth very well with clean water 3-4 times after every eating.

Have one day fast in a month giving rest to your stomach taking lemon water or plane drinking water with or without honey throughout the day and fruits in the evening. Or otherwise skip one meal once a week taking only fruits & juice or soups in the dinner.

Be optimistic and have always positive thinking. Be kind to others. Do not forget to thank for any favour to you or to say sorry for any mistake. Have a nature of Forget any mis-happenings and forgive others for their fault.

Put paintings with good-slogans in your living room and kitchen with quote like "Take Food like Medicines otherwise have to take medicines like food" "We have come empty hand and will go empty hand- our good work will only be remembered " " have your behaviour to others as you like for yourself" " Go or not to go-better go; Eat or not to eat-better not to eat" "Only Diet can heal us or will make us sick" etc.

After the age of 30 years, have a full body-check-up and comprehensive blood & urine-test which can give you result of well-functioning of all body parts including kidney-lever-lungs-heart-eyes; blood-sugar- blood-pressure- eye-pressure etc. once a year. Keep digital good quality blood-pressure and blood-sugar testing machine at home and check weekly after the age of 40 years. Do not ignore any symptoms of health problem. Prefer naturopathy- acupressure- physiotherapy if applicable- then homeopathy then Ayurvedic or Unani or Chinese or Japanese healing system & medicines – then allopathy chemical medicines be the last option. In case of any emergency never delay consulting your doctor and going to the hospital.

Donate 1% or 2% of your annual income to some charity for philanthropic purpose of your interest. Volunteer your time & expertise, if available, for some charitable purpose. Never forget to console your family & friends in case of their trouble and visiting any sick member you know.

During your week ends and once in a year for 8 to 10 days with your family, have some fun by going to tourist places near you or theatre or picnic or whatever suitable & convenient to you. It will re-energise you.

CHAPTER 3

Know about your important Organs of the body and how to keep them healthy to make you disease free

Our body is also like a machine. There are many organs in our body like different parts of a machine. We should know about their functions and importance. By keeping them all in good working condition, disease free, our whole body will remail disease free. All organs are related to each other and effects on other part of the body.

3.1. Heart

Heart, the main organ in our cardiovascular system, is vital for our life. Its parts work together to move blood through our body in a coordinated way. It constantly sends oxygen to our cells and takes away waste.

The essential functions of heart are: 1. pumping oxygenated blood to body tissues, 2. receiving deoxygenated blood, 3. maintaining blood pressure, 4. routing blood through the lungs for oxygenation, 5. regulating blood flow by adjusting heart rate, 6. providing nutrients to its tissues through coronary circulation.

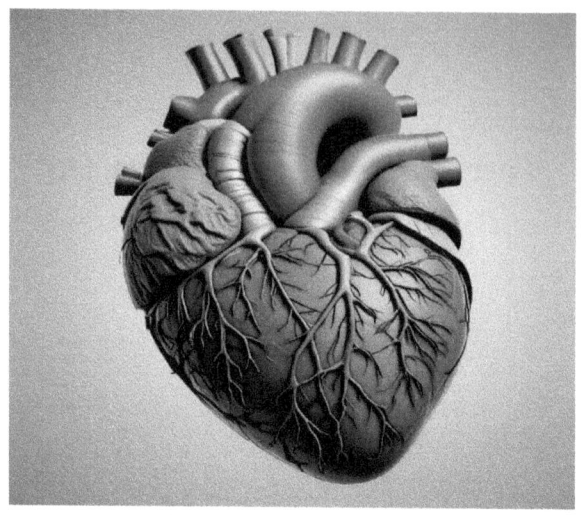

The heart move blood throughout our body. Blood brings oxygen and nutrients to our cells. It also takes away carbon dioxide and other waste so other organs can dispose of them. The heart also Controls the rhythm and speed of our heart rate and maintains our blood pressure.

The heart works with Nervous system, which helps control our heart rate. It sends signals that tell the heart to beat slower during rest and faster during stress. The Endocrine system sends out hormones. These hormones tell our blood vessels to constrict or relax, which affects our blood pressure. Hormones from our thyroid gland can also tell our heart to beat faster or slower.

Heart disease is the leading cause of death for both men and women in the world. To prevent heart disease, we must -

- Eat a heart-healthy diet
- Get active

- Stay at a healthy weight
- Quit smoking and stay away from second-hand smoke
- Control our cholesterol, blood glucose (sugar), and blood pressure
- Quit Alcohol or Drink alcohol only in moderation
- Manage stress Be Positive Trust God
- Get enough sleep

How to Keep Heart Healthy:

1. Control food quantity: How much you eat is just as important as what you eat. As mentioned in chapter one, eat that much quantity of food so that you feel full hunger at the time of our next food time. To control portion, keep less cooked grains and increase vegetables, sprouted items, salads & fruits etc. in our daily diet.

2. Eat more fibre. Eat vegetables, fruits, beans, onion, cucumber, salads, tomato and cabbage to add fibre to our diet. Vegetables and fruits are good sources of fibre, vitamins and minerals. They are low in calories and rich in fibre. Vegetables and fruits, like other plants or plant-based foods, contain substances that may help prevent heart disease. Eating more fruits and vegetables also may help you eat less high calorie food.

3. Choose whole grains: Whole grains are good sources of fiber and other nutrients that play roles in heart's good health and controlling blood pressure

4. Limit unhealthy fats: Limit the amount of saturated and trans fats you eat. This helps lower our blood

cholesterol and lower our risk of a common heart condition called coronary artery disease. A high blood cholesterol level can lead to a buildup of plaques in the arteries, called atherosclerosis. And that can raise the risk of heart attack and stroke. Limit or avoid foods like pizza, burgers, processed & packed or canned foods, and creamy sauces or gravy etc. It is my experience in own life that taking 3-4 cloves of garlic early in the morning keeps cholesterol level down and reduces blood thickness for easy flow, reducing workload of the heart.

5. Choose low-fat protein sources: Legumes — beans, peas and lentils — also are good low-fat sources of protein. They contain no cholesterol, making them good substitutes for meat. Eating plant protein instead of animal protein lowers the amounts of fat and cholesterol you take in. It also boosts how much fibre you get.

6. Limit and reduce sodium and salt: Sodium is a mineral. It's found naturally in some foods, such as celery or milk. Food makers add sodium to processed foods, such as bread and soup. Eating foods with lots of added sodium can lead to high blood pressure. So can using table salt, which contains sodium.

7. Healthy daily menus: Plan daily menus using the tips listed above. When you choose foods for each meal and snack, focus on vegetables, fruits, and whole grains. Choose lean proteins and healthy fats and limit salty foods. Watch our portion sizes and add variety to our menu choices.

8. Other precautions to keep heart healthy is to lose weight, stop or control smoking & alcohol consumption.

These creates significant risks to heart attacks and other heart diseases.

3.2. Lungs

Lungs is another very important organ linked to heart. Lungs provide oxygen to every cell in our body. When we breathe in air, oxygen moves into our bloodstream. The blood takes it to the cells around our body. At each cell, oxygen is exchanged for a waste gas called carbon dioxide. Our bloodstream then carries carbon dioxide back to our lungs. It leaves our body when you breathe out.

This is an automatic process starting at birth till we die. The cycle happens eight to 16 times every minute.

Thus, the most important function of the lungs is to take oxygen from the environment and transfer it to the bloodstream. The lungs are the major organ of the respiratory system as is the heart, which helps provide the body with a continuous supply of oxygen.

When we inhale through our nose or mouth, air travels down our pharynx (back of our throat), passes through our larynx (voice box) and into our trachea (windpipe).

For our lungs to perform their best, our air-ways need to be open when you inhale and when you exhale. They also need to be free from inflammation (swelling) and abnormal amounts of mucus.

After absorbing oxygen, the blood leaves our lungs and is carried to our heart. From there, it's pumped through our body to provide oxygen to every cells of our tissues and organs. When cells use oxygen, they produce carbon dioxide and transfer it to our blood. The bloodstream carries the carbon dioxide back to our lungs. When we exhale, we remove the carbon dioxide out.

The respiratory system prevents harmful substances from entering our lungs by using:

Small hairs in our nose that act as an air-cleaning system and help filter out large particles.

Mucus produced in our trachea and bronchial tubes to keep air passages moist and help catch dust, bacteria and other substances.

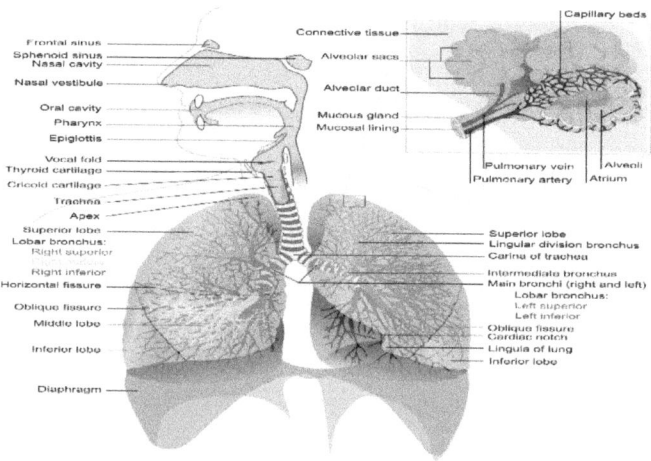

The sweeping motion of cilia (small hairs in our respiratory tract) to keep air passages clean. One of the reasons that cigarette smoke is dangerous is that it stops cilia from working properly.

There are many things you can do to keep our lungs healthy or to help manage lung conditions.

1. Breath fresh air free from pollution, dust, smoke, bad-smell etc. Use hygienic cotton masks covering our nose & mouth, if the air is polluted. Make sure that the places where you live and work are well ventilated for fresh air and cleaned regularly to prevent the buildup of allergens.
2. Breath with nose, avoid breathing by mouth.
3. In office, the workplace should have proper fresh-air ventilation. In our home and sleeping room too, should have windows or ventilators for fresh air flow for good health of the lungs.
4. Stop smoking & vaping or second-hand smoking
5. Try to reach and maintain a healthy weight. People with obesity have less space for lung expansion.
6. Exercise regularly. Yoga is more beneficial for lungs. Physical activity can help strengthen our heart and lungs, so they work more efficiently. Physical activity may also reduce our risk of lung injury or disease.
7. Eat healthy foods in moderation. Some best food items for healthy lungs are Beets and beet greens, peppers, apple, pumpkin, turmeric, garlic, onion, tomato, berries, cabbage, yogurt, barley, lentils etc.
8. Stay hydrated, unless our provider gives you a limit on how much liquid you can drink.
9. Limit our exposure to people who are sick having respiratory diseases or use good masks when you go near to them.
10. Laughing: Laughing is the best remedy for healthy lungs. It is a great exercise to work the

abdominal muscles and increase lung capacity. It also clears out our lungs by forcing enough stale air out that allows fresh air to enter into more areas of the lung. Laughter provides longer exhalations, thus expelling residual air from the lungs and enriching the blood with ample supplies of oxygen. As one breathes deeply during a hearty laugh, lungs are saturated with oxygenated blood, we may cough, sputter or spit phlegm, due to loosening up of mucus in our respiratory system and getting a good fresh cleaning.

Join or organize a laughter's club for healthy lungs in our town or city or village.

11. Do deep breathing: Deep breathing can help you get closer to reaching our lungs' full capacity. Take deep breath, keep it for some time as much as you can and then exhale. Expand our chest to allow air to fill our lungs. As you slowly inhale, consciously expand our belly with awareness of lowering the diaphragm. Next, expand our ribs, allowing them to float open like wings. Finally, allow the upper chest to expand and lift. Then exhale as completely as possible by letting the chest fall, and then contracting the ribs and, finally, bringing our stomach muscles in and up to lift the diaphragm and expel the last bit of air.

12. Counting' our breaths

You can also increase our lung capacity by increasing the length of our inhalations and exhalations. Start by counting how long a natural breath takes. If it takes to the count of five to inhale, it should take to the count of five to exhale. Try to keep them to an equal length.

Once you've discovered the count for our average breath, add one more count to each inhale and exhale until you can comfortably extend the length of time it takes to fill and empty our lungs.

3.3. Kidney

The kidneys are two bean-shaped organs in the renal system. They are one of main filter system of our body. They help the body pass waste as urine. They also help filter blood before sending it back to the heart.

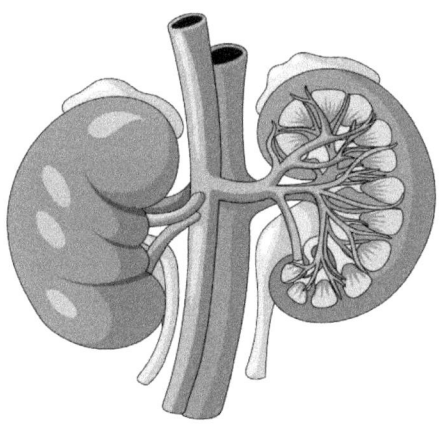

The kidneys perform many crucial functions, including:

- maintaining overall fluid balance
- regulating and filtering minerals from blood

- filtering waste materials from food, medications, and toxic substances
- creating hormones that help produce red blood cells, promote bone health, and regulate blood pressure

Kidney – the filter system of our body: The main job of the kidneys is to remove waste from the blood and return the cleaned blood back to the heart. Each minute about one litre of blood – one-fifth of all the blood pumped by the heart – enters the kidneys through the renal arteries. After the blood is cleaned, it flows back into the body through the renal veins.

Each kidney contains about one million tiny units called nephrons. Each nephron is made up of a very small filter, called a glomerulus, which is attached to a tubule. As blood passes through the nephron, fluid and waste products are filtered out. Much of the fluid is then returned to the blood, while the waste products are concentrated in any extra fluid as urine (wee).

The urine flows through a tube called the ureter into the bladder. Urine passes from the bladder out of the body through a tube called the urethra. The kidney usually makes one to two litres of urine every day depending on our build, how much you drink, the temperature and the amount of exercise you do.

As well as filtering the blood, kidneys make and regulate important hormones in the body that help to control blood pressure, red blood cell production and calcium uptake from the intestine. They maintain body fluid at the correct levels for the body to function. They control body chemistry by regulating the amount of salt, water and other chemicals moving around the body.

To keep kidneys healthy: The kidneys are important organs that affect many other body parts, including the heart. Steps to keep them working efficiently are_

Drink enough water: Enough water is must to keep our kidney function well and having all its filtration parts managed taking out toxins. The test is colour of your urine. If you have taken enough water, the urine will be very light yellow.

Make healthy food choices: For good health of our kidney, heart and lungs, choose foods that are healthy for our entire body: fresh fruits, fresh or frozen vegetables, whole grains, and low-fat or fat-free dairy products. Cut down on salt, added sugars and packaged food items.

Avoid extra salt: Eating a lot of salty foods can disrupt the balance of minerals in the blood. This can make it harder for the kidneys to work properly. Try swapping out processed foods — which usually have a lot of added salt — for whole foods, such as fresh fruits and vegetables, lean cuts of meat, nuts

Exercise: High blood pressure is a known risk factor for chronic kidney disease. Keep blood pressure normal. Regular exercise, even for just 20 minutes a day, can help reduce blood pressure, besides taking other measures to control blood pressure.

Diabetes: Diabetes is another very risk factor damaging the Kidneys. Hence control our blood sugar to keep kidneys healthy and function well.

Obesity: Overweight and fatness is also dangerous for damaging kidneys. Keep our weight under control by reducing oily food, junk food and diet control

3.4. Lever

The liver is another main organ in the body supporting detoxification processes and has many other critical jobs. Our environment and lifestyle choices greatly affect how well and efficiently the liver carries out its work. Adopting a healthy lifestyle is one of the biggest drivers to preventing liver disease.

Major functions of the liver are:

The liver regulates most chemical levels in the blood and excretes a product called bile. This helps carry away waste products from the liver. All the blood leaving the stomach and intestines passes through the liver. The liver processes this blood and breaks down, balances, and creates the nutrients and also metabolizes drugs into forms that are easier to use for the rest of the body or that are nontoxic. More than 500 vital functions have been identified with the liver.

Some of the more well-known functions include the following:

Production of bile, which helps carry away waste and break down fats in the small intestine during digestion

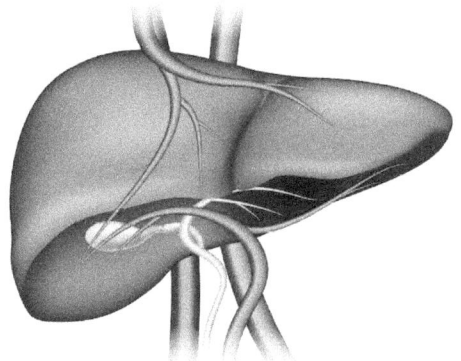

Production of certain proteins for blood plasma

Production of cholesterol and special proteins to help carry fats through the body

Conversion of excess glucose into glycogen for storage (glycogen can later be converted back to glucose for energy) and to balance and make glucose as needed

Regulation of blood levels of amino acids, which form the building blocks of proteins

Processing of haemoglobin for use of its iron content (the liver stores iron)

Conversion of poisonous ammonia to urea (urea is an end product of protein metabolism and is excreted in the urine)

Clearing the blood of drugs and other poisonous substances

Regulating blood clotting

Resisting infections by making immune factors and removing bacteria from the bloodstream

Clearance of bilirubin, also from red blood cells. If there is an accumulation of bilirubin, the skin and eyes turn yellow.

When the liver has broken down harmful substances, its by-products are excreted into the bile or blood. Bile by-products enter the intestine and leave the body in the form of feces. Blood by-products are filtered out by the kidneys and leave the body in the form of urine.

Knowing liver is so important for our good health, we must take steps to keep liver heathy

1. Eat simple homemade food of whole grains with less oils and spices and having enough fibre like green vegetables, nuts, beans, fruits, salads, sprouted food items etc.

    Eating a diet rich in fibre and simple food (without fried in oil and mixed with spices) with lots of salad etc. is linked to a lower risk of causing liver-disease and developing fatty liver. Fiber promotes a healthy weight and balanced energy levels, whereas excess energy (or calories) is the main driver of fat buildup in liver cells.

2. Maintain your weight & diet to maintain your liver: Over-weight and obesity leads to fatty lever and other lever problems. Hence by controlling the quality and quantity of diet, not making stomach a dustbin sending food whenever you like or get, avoiding junk food, leaving sugar and its products

as explained in chapter one and with regular exercise you can maintain a healthy weight and will be free from all problems and disease of liver. Exercise, physical work, walking, jogging and yoga are very good for our health including the healthy liver. Make it in your daily routine.

3. Quit or control alcohol/wine/liquor and smoking, if you want liver be always in healthy condition and do all its functions as desired, quit or control taking wine/alcohol/smoking or other forms of such drinks or drugs which are very dangerous to liver.

The body treats alcohol and smoke as a toxin, and it's the liver's job to neutralize the toxin. And while it can do that, prolonged, excessive alcohol intake damage the liver and is the cause of alcoholic fatty liver disease. So please stop taking alcohol or limit it very much with your willpower & determination.

4. Have sufficient sleep and Control stress, tension and anxiety: Chronic stress/tension/anxiety negatively impacts liver function, may be physical or emotional—immune function is interrupted and can lead to inflammation of the liver. In addition, hormone shifts interfere with blood flow to the liver, damaging cells.

Taking 7 to 8 hours of uninterrupted sleep is also very necessary for a healthy liver. When you go to bed, forget all your worries for few hours, wash your feet with warm water, have a prayer on your bed to God for a meaningful day & tomorrow and sleep stress-free. Good diet, eating at least 2 hours before going to bed, daily exercise, enjoying free time before sleeping, may lead to a good sleep. Liver goes on working when you are sleeping so improving sleep and sleep quality is a great way to support your liver.

5. Drink enough water: Dehydration and drinking less water (less than 2 to 4 litres of water in a day as per the age & season) damages most of the organs of the body including liver. As suggested earlier take 2 to 3 glasses of water early morning before going to toilet, one glass before and after breakfast, one glass of water before and after lunch and dinner, two glasses at interval in the afternoon & juice in the evening and one glass of hot milk with turmeric before going to bed can maintain the body hydrated and safe.

3.5. Thyroid

The thyroid gland is a vital endocrine (hormone-producing) gland. It plays a major role in chemical reactions in the body (our metabolism), as well as our growth and development. It helps to regulate many body functions by constantly releasing a certain amount of thyroid hormones into the bloodstream.

The thyroid gland produces three hormones: Triiodothyronine, also known as T3; Tetraiodothyronine, also called thyroxine or T4 and Calcitonin

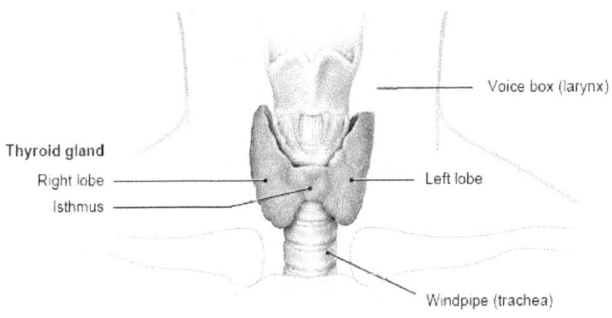

Iodine is one of the main building blocks of both hormones. Our bodies can't produce this trace element, so we need to get enough of it in our diet. Iodine is absorbed into our bloodstream from food in our bowel. It is then carried to the thyroid gland, where it is eventually used to make thyroid hormones.

What to do for maintaining the Thyroid healthy:

Our diet: Stick to a diet that is low in sugar. Excessive sugar can lead to inflammation, which can worsen the symptoms of an underactive thyroid Take food rich in nutrients essential for thyroid health. Incorporate iodine-rich foods like seaweed, fish, dairy, and iodized salt. Selenium from nuts, seeds, and legumes supports thyroid function, while zinc from whole grains, nuts, and lean meats aids in hormone production. It is sad that some vegetables like cabbage and broccoli can interfere with thyroid hormone production, so limit there use in your food.

No to processed foods: Processed foods often contain additives that can disrupt thyroid function. Minimize intake of refined sugars, high-fat foods, and artificial additives. Instead, opt for whole foods to support a healthy thyroid.

Control stress: It's been shown that stress can cause thyroid hormone resistance. Chronic stress can negatively impact thyroid function. Engage in stress-relieving activities like yoga, meditation, deep breathing exercises or hobbies to maintain healthy cortisol levels and support your thyroid.

Physical Exercise & Yoga: Physical exercise, physically be active and yoga improves metabolism and helps regulate hormone levels. Aim for a balanced exercise routine that includes cardiovascular workouts, strength training and flexibility exercises for optimal thyroid health.

Maintain a healthy body weight. The higher your body weight, the more thyroid hormone your body will require. Do sufficient physical activity daily to control getting overweight.

Sufficient sleep: Good sleep is very important for overall health, including thyroid function. Aim for 7 to 9 hours of sleep each night to support hormone production and regulate metabolism.

Take care of pollution & toxins: Toxins in the environment, such as pollutants, chemicals and heavy metals, can interfere with thyroid function. Minimize exposure by using masks covering nose & mouth and other natural cleaning products, filtering drinking water and being mindful of environmental pollutants.

Do regular check-ups: Time to time check-ups is essential for early detection of any potential thyroid issues. If you have symptoms of an overactive or underactive thyroid, have a test—a blood test measuring your hormone levels to check for issues or abnormalities.

3.6. Brain

Brain is an essential organ that controls many body functions. Your brain receives and interprets all the sensory information you encounter, like sights, sounds, smells and tastes. Your brain has many complex parts that work together to help you function.

Healthy lifestyle choices and managing chronic health conditions can help keep your brain healthy.

Your brain enables:

- Thoughts and decisions.
- Memories and emotions.
- Movements (motor function), balance and coordination.
- Perception of various sensations including pain.
- Automatic behaviour such as breathing, heart rate, sleep and temperature control.
- Regulation of organ function.

Speech and language functions

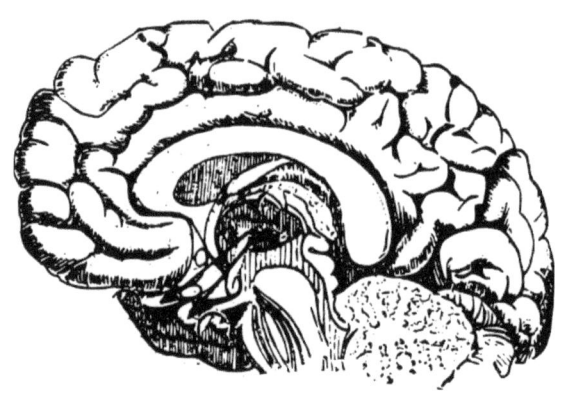

Maintaining Your Brain Health

Manage blood sugar, blood pressure and Cholesterol: The health of your arteries and veins is important to your heart health but it is also critical for brain health. Get your blood pressure, blood sugar and cholesterol checked regularly and take steps to keep your numbers within a normal range.

Be physically active and do regular exercise: Exercise has many known benefits, and regular physical activity also benefits the brain. Also, any mentally stimulating activity should help to build up your brain.

Diet: Your diet plays a large role in your brain health. Consider following a Mediterranean diet, which emphasizes plant-based foods, whole grains, fish and healthy fats, such as olive oil.

Quit smoking and avoid tobacco in all its forms. Excessive drinking is a major risk factor for dementia. If you choose to drink, limit yourself be in a safe health

Protect your head: Moderate to severe head injuries may harm brain, even without diagnosed concussions, increase the risk of cognitive impairment. Always use helmets when using two-wheelers and follow traffic rules while driving. Also, in home, bathroom & workplace be cautious of slippery surfaces not to get fall.

Maintain a healthy weight: Obesity is harmful for health and cause of many diseases, also affecting brain-health.

Get enough sleep: Sleep plays an important role in your brain health. Some theories state that sleep helps clear abnormal proteins in your brain and consolidates memories, which boosts your overall memory and brain health.

Stay engaged: Your brain is like a muscle — you need to use it or lose it. There are many things that you can do to keep your brain in shape, such as doing crossword puzzles or Sudoku, reading, playing cards or putting together a jigsaw puzzle.

Social engagement and involvement in charitable works keeps us engaged, happy and helps ward off depression and stress, which can contribute to memory loss. Look for opportunities to connect with charities, volunteering, laughter's' club, friends and others.

3.7. Stomach & Digestive System

The digestive system breaks down food and liquid into their chemical components—carbohydrates, fats, proteins, vitamins, and minerals—so the body can absorb these nutrients, use them for energy, and build or repair cells.

Many organs make up the digestive system. Digestion begins the moment food is chewed and travels from the mouth, down the oesophagus, and into the stomach. Once in the stomach, food is mixed with digestive enzymes and then slowly emptied into the small intestine, which further breaks down food, absorbs nutrients, and sends them into bloodstream.

The remaining watery food residue moves into your large intestine (the colon). As undigested food passes through it, bacteria feed off the remnants. The wall of the large intestine soaks up most of the remaining water.

Other organs also contribute to the digestive process. The liver produces bile, a brownish-yellow liquid that helps to digest fat. Bile is stored until needed in the gallbladder. The pancreas works with the small intestine to produce enzymes needed to help digest proteins, fats, and carbohydrates

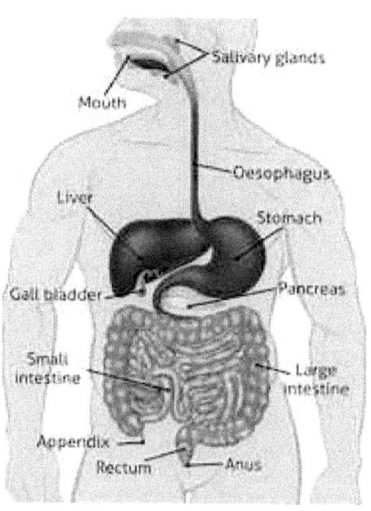

Any undigested food that remains is expelled by a highly efficient disposal system involving the rectum and anus.

To maintain healthy stomach and the good digestive system, the required measures are:

Take right foods to help your digestion: Take food filled up with fibre and easy to digest which avoid constipation. A diet rich in fibre can help digestion and prevent constipation. Such as salads, sprouted food items, wholemeal bread, brown rice, fruit and veg, beans, oats, etc.

Do not eat without hunger: Hunger is the signal that your stomach and digestive system is ready. Never eat without hunger. Skip meal if you are not hungry. Do not make stomach a dustbin, sending food whenever & whatever you get.

Drink plenty of fluids to aid digestion: It is important to keep drinking, especially water. It encourages the passage of waste through your digestive system and helps soften poo. Fibre acts like a sponge, absorbing water. Without fluid, the fibre cannot do its job, and you'll get constipation. Drink 3 to 4 litres of fluid a day in form of plain water 2-3 litre and rest in form of juice or milk etc. Avoid caffeine drinks as they can cause heartburn.

Cut down on fat for a healthy gut: Fatty foods, such as chips, burgers, pizza and fried foods, are harder to digest and can cause constipation, stomach pain and heartburn. Avoid oily or greasy fried foods to ease your stomach's workload. Spicy foods may give you heartburn, stomach pain or diarrhoea, control them. If you already have a problem like heartburn or an irritable bowel, avoid them completely.

Avoid cold-drinks, alcohol, coffee, tea, fizzy drinks: These drinks are acidic and cause problems to digestive system & stomach. Drinks with caffeine, such as coffee, colas, tea and some fizzy drinks, boost acid in the stomach, leading to heartburn. Fizzy drinks in general tend to bloat the tummy, which can also lead to heartburn. To make digestive problems less likely, choose drinks that are not fizzy and do not contain caffeine, such as herbal teas, milk and plain water.

3.8. Eyes

Eyes are our most important organ helping us to see the world and do all our daily living activities & work smoothly. Therefore, it is very important to keep your eyes and vision in good condition.

Eye Problems: Refraction error, cataract, glaucoma, blurry vision, spots, glare at night, double vision, flashing lights, watering eyes, night blindness etc.- these are common eye complaints. Each could be an early sign of disease.

Splashing fresh clean normal water into your open eyes with mouth full of water during teeth-brush is a healthy habit, which I do and found its great benefit, Other than that to keep your eyes in good health and vision perfect

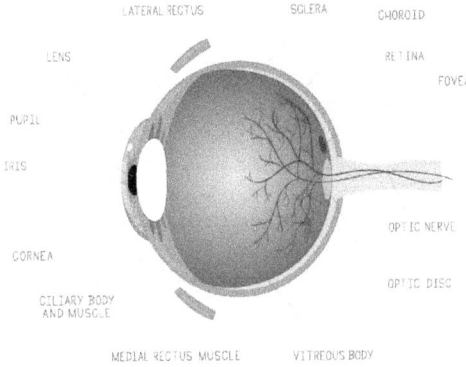

follow the tips given below:

1. Eat Well: Good eye health starts with the food on your plate. Nutrients like omega-3 fatty acids, lutein, zinc, and vitamins C and E might help ward off age-related vision problems like macular degeneration and cataracts.

Vitamin A plays an important role in your vision. To see the full spectrum of light, your eye needs to produce certain pigments for your retina to work properly. Vitamin A deficiency stops the production of these pigments, leading to night blindness. Your eye also needs vitamin A to nourish other parts of your eye, including the cornea. Without enough vitamin A, your eyes cannot produce enough moisture to keep them properly lubricated.

To get them, fill your plate with:

- Green leafy vegetables like spinach, kale, and collards in your daily diet is essential for proper vision.

- Carrot, sweet potato, pumpkins are rich in vitamin A supporting good eye health.
- Salmon, tuna, and other oily fish
- Eggs, nuts, beans, and other nonmeat protein sources
- Oranges and other citrus fruits or fresh juices

A well-balanced diet also helps you stay at a healthy weight. That lowers your odds of obesity and related diseases like type 2 diabetes, which is the leading cause of blindness in adults.

Diabetes affects retina of the eyes and is responsible for diabetic retinopathy, leading to permanent blindness if not detected and treated on time. Hence, avoid sugar and sugar products, junk food, packaged food with added sugar, more starchy food, have healthy lifestyle mentioned in chapter one and eliminate all causes of getting diabetes.

2. Quit Smoking: It makes you more likely to get cataracts, damage to your optic nerve, and macular degeneration, among many other medical problems. If you've tried to kick the habit before only to start again, keep at it. The more times you try to quit, the more likely you are to succeed. Ask your doctor for help.

3. Wear Sunglasses: The right pair of shades will help protect your eyes from the sun's ultraviolet (UV) rays. Too much UV exposure boosts your chances of cataracts and macular degeneration.

If you wear contact lenses, some offer UV protection. It's still a good idea to wear sunglasses for an extra layer.

4. Use Safety Eyewear: If you use hazardous or airborne materials on the job or at home, wear safety glasses or protective goggles. Sports like ice hockey, racquetball, and lacrosse can also lead to eye injury. Wear eye protection. Helmets with protective face masks or sports goggles with polycarbonate lenses will shield your eyes.

5. Look Away From the Computer Screen: Staring at a computer or phone screen for too long can cause: Eyestrain; Blurry vision; Trouble focusing at a distance; Dry eyes; Headaches; Neck, back, and shoulder pain

To protect your eyes: Make sure your glasses or contacts prescription is up to date and good for looking at a computer screen. If your eye strain won't go away, talk to your doctor about computer glasses. Move the screen so your eyes are level with the top of the monitor. That lets you look slightly down at the screen. Try to avoid glare from windows and lights. Use an anti-glare screen if needed. Choose a comfortable, supportive chair. Position it so that your feet are flat on the floor. Rest your eyes every 20 minutes. Look 20 feet away for 20 seconds. Get up at least every 2 hours and take a 15-minute break.

6. Visit Your Eye Doctor Regularly: Everyone needs a regular eye exam, even young children. It helps protect your sight and lets you see your best. Eye exams can also find diseases, like glaucoma, that have no symptoms. It's important to spot them early on, when they're easier to treat.

3.9. Ear

Ears are another important organ of our body which helps us to hear and get connected to people easily & smoothly and makes our life happier by enjoying music.

To keep our ears in good condition and to avoid hearing loss untimely take the following steps: -

1. Clean your ears the right way: Earwax isn't dirty or unhealthy. In fact, it's the opposite. Earwax helps ward off fungal infections and bacteria. And it helps keep out tiny particles that can cause damage to your eardrum. That includes things like dust and hair. Earwax is your body's built-in system for cleaning your ears and a natural moisturizer."

If you have a build-up of earwax that's blocking your hearing or creating a muffled sound, see a healthcare provider to have it removed. Don't try to remove it on your own. If you have pierced ears, clean your earrings and earlobes regularly with rubbing alcohol.

ANATOMY OF THE EAR

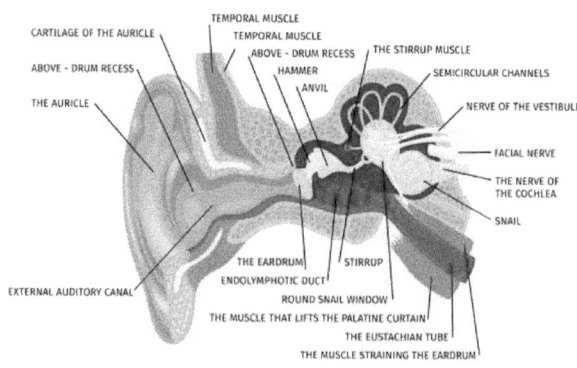

2. Wear Earplugs Around Loud Noises: Loud noises such as those emitted by power tools, concerts, lawnmowers, firearms, and aircraft can all gradually lead to hearing loss, especially if you are exposed to these noises on a regular basis. Wear earplugs in environments that expose you to loud noises to protect your ears and reduce your risk of hearing loss. Your employer or otolaryngologist (ear, nose, and throat doctor) can recommend the best earplugs for you based on your environment.

3. Turn Down the Volume: Listening to loud music can damage your hearing, especially when using earbuds that sit directly next to your eardrum. Keep the volume turned down when watching television or listening to music in your home or vehicle and consider using over-the-ear headphones instead of earbuds, which place more distance between your eardrums and noise from portable devices.

Concerts and clubs may be extremely fun, but they also have the potential to cause temporary or permanent hearing loss. When attending loud events such as these, take frequent breaks by stepping outside or going somewhere to separate yourself from the noise, even if just for five minutes. After the event has ended, try to spend time in a quiet environment for at least one day to allow your ears to rest and recover.

4. Stop Using Cotton Swabs: People have been using cotton swabs for decades to remove earwax buildup from the inside of their ears, but researchers have found that cotton swabs may actually do more harm than good. The cotton swabs can push earwax deeper into the ear canal

to damage the eardrum and ear canal to increase the risk for hearing problems.

Your doctor may recommend using a soft, damp tool to clean the opening of your ear canal or using an approved ear wax removal solution that softens the wax so it can flow more easily out of your ear canal.

5. Keep safe Ears from water: Swimming and bathing can result in water entering your ear canal, which can be risky for your hearing and ear health if the water contains harmful bacteria or sits in your ear canal for a long period. Tilt your head to the side after bathing or swimming to help excess water drain out of your ears, or use a small, soft towel to soak up excess water in your ears.

If you swim regularly, consider buying earplugs specially designed for swimmers that prevent water from entering your ear canal. Your otolaryngologist may also order custom-fit earplugs that fit snugly and comfortably inside your ears.

6. Use Medications Properly as Directed: Hearing loss is a side effect of many different medications. Drug-induced hearing loss is known as ototoxicity, which may occur in those who use specific drugs in high doses or for a long period. Take them responsibly and properly as directed. You may also want to ask your doctor about other treatments for your health condition that won't increase your risk for hearing loss.

7. Stay Physically Active: Exercising regularly promotes good blood flow and circulation, which helps blood and oxygen reach your ears to keep them in optimal health.

Make exercise a priority and aim to be active on most days of the week to protect your hearing and ear health. The best way to stay engaged with an exercise routine is to do activities you truly enjoy. Dance, go for daily walks, or play outdoor games with your family.

8. Manage and Reduce Stress: Stress increases your body's production of cortisol and adrenaline, which are stress hormones released as a fight-or-flight response to potential threats. These hormones can temporarily affect your hearing, which is completely normal. However, long-term stress can lead to elevated levels of these hormones, which increases the risk of permanent hearing loss.

Find effective ways to manage and reduce stress, as chronic stress can lead to a large number of health problems in addition to hearing loss. Listen to soothing music, exercise daily, or find other outlets that allow you to release pent-up stress and anxiety. You may also want to focus on eliminating certain stressors from your life that are causing you to experience chronic stress.

9. Know the Warning Signs of Hearing Damage: Ringing in the ears, dizziness, muffled sound in the ears, and loss of balance are common signs of early or temporary hearing damage. If you are in an environment with loud noises and start to experience any signs of hearing loss, remove yourself from the situation as soon as possible to protect your hearing. You may also want to visit your otolaryngologist for a hearing appointment to confirm whether or not you are developing hearing loss.

10. Stop Smoking, and Don't Start: Smoking reduces your blood oxygen levels and narrows blood vessels all

throughout the body, including those Smoking may irritates and blocks the Eustachian tubes, which connect the middle ears to the back of the throat and are responsible for draining fluid and maintaining air pressure in the ears. Smoking also interferes with nerves in the ear to make you more sensitive to loud noises and increase your risk for hearing loss.

If you're a smoker, take steps to quit as soon as possible to prevent hearing loss. If you don't smoke, don't start, as nicotine is a habit-forming substance that can lead to a harmful, long-term habit.

11. Keep your ears safe from injury: Some activities can put your ears at risk for injury. Minimize your potential by: Wearing a helmet when you bike, ski or participate in any other activity that puts you at risk for head and ear injuries.

Learning proper underwater techniques to avoid potentially damaging changes in pressure inside your ears when scuba diving.

Swallowing and yawning frequently when flying in an airplane, particularly when the plane is landing. That helps equalize pressure in your ears. Consider getting earplugs with special filters designed for air travel.

12. Visit Your Doctor Regularly for Checkups: Many otolaryngologists recommend getting your hearing tested every three to five years if you are between the ages of 18 and 40. Your doctor may recommend being screened more frequently if you have started to experience some degree of hearing loss or have a medical

condition such as an autoimmune disorder or meningitis that may lead to hearing loss.

3.10. Teeth & Gums

Without teeth we cannot imagine having happier life and enjoying the food. Good, shining, white teeth are making our personality too. To keep our teeth and gums healthy please follow the tips given below:

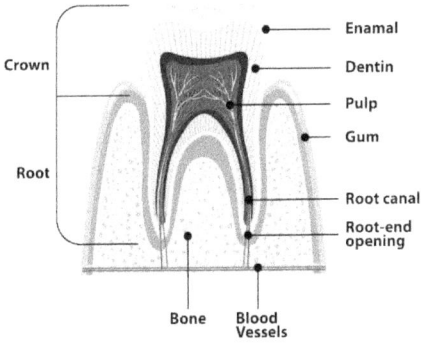

1. Brushing and flossing your teeth are not hard to do but do it correctly to help prevent gum disease and tooth loss. Gum disease is caused by bacteria found in plaque and tartar. Plaque is a sticky film that forms on the teeth. It is mostly made up of bacteria, mucus, food, and other particles. When plaque isn't removed, it hardens into tartar, which gives a home to bacteria. Bacteria in plaque and tartar cause inflammation of the gums, called gingivitis.

Symptoms of periodontal disease often appear when the condition is advanced. Symptoms are: Bad breath that lasts, Red, swollen, sore gums; Gums that bleed easily, Gums that pull away from the teeth (receding gums); Pain when chewing; Loose or sensitive teeth

Good oral hygiene, such as brushing and flossing at least twice every day, can help prevent gum infections, cavities, and tooth loss. Having your teeth cleaned and checked by a dentist or dental hygienist at least once a year also is important.

To brush correctly:

- Brush in the morning and before going to sleep.
- Use a soft-bristled brush and toothpaste that contains fluoride. If you can afford the cost, buy and use an electric toothbrush.
- Place your toothbrush at a 45° angle against your gums and brush each tooth 15 to 20 times.
- Move the brush gently, using short strokes. Don't scrub.
- Brush the outer tooth surfaces using short, back-and-forth strokes.
- Brush the inner upper front teeth by brushing vertically against them using short, downward strokes. Use short, upward strokes for lower inside teeth.
- Brush the chewing surfaces of the teeth with short, back-and-forth strokes. Replace your toothbrush when it's worn or frayed about every 3 or 4 months, experts say. You should also get a new toothbrush

after you have had a cold, strep throat, or similar illness.
- Don't cover your toothbrush or store it in a closed container. This can encourage growth of microorganisms.

Flossing helps to remove plaque and food particles that are stuck between your teeth and under your gums. To floss correctly:

- Cut off about 18 inches of floss and hold it tightly between your thumbs and forefingers. Place it between your teeth and gently slide it up and down.
- When the floss reaches the gum line, curve it around 1 tooth in a C shape. Gently rub the side of the tooth, moving the floss with up-and-down motions, making sure to go below the gumline. Repeat this method on the rest of your teeth. Remember to floss the back side of your back teeth.

Quit Tobacco: Tobacco use can cause many oral health problems, including:

- Gum disease: Smoking is a leading cause of gum disease, which can damage the bone that supports your teeth. Gum disease can lead to tooth loss.
- Tooth decay: Tobacco use can cause tooth decay.
- Tooth staining: Nicotine and tar in tobacco can stain teeth yellow or brown.
- Mouth cancer: Smoking is a leading cause of mouth cancer.

- Dry socket: Smokers are more likely to develop dry socket after a tooth extraction. Dry socket is a painful condition that occurs when the blood clot at the extraction site doesn't form properly.
- Leucoplakia: Smokeless tobacco use can cause white or gray patches to form in the mouth, which can lead to cancer.
- Bad breath: Smoking can cause bad breath, also known as halitosis.
- Decreased taste: Smoking can cause a loss of taste.

Vaping can also cause oral health problems, including gum disease, cavities, and tooth damage.

Quit Smoking: The gums are affected because smoking causes a lack of oxygen in the bloodstream, so the infected gums don't heal. Smoking causes people to have more dental plaque and causes gum disease to get worse more quickly than in non-smokers. Gum disease is still the most common cause of tooth loss in adults.

Eat proper food for better health of teeth & gum: The foods you eat help lead to tooth decay when they combine with bacteria in your mouth. To protect your teeth:

- Have plenty of calcium-rich foods, such as milk, yogurt, cheese, canned fish, almonds, beans, green leafy vegetables, and calcium-fortified orange juice. Calcium maintains the bone the tooth roots are embedded in.
- Limit sugary foods and drinks. Stay away from sugar, sugar products and sticky sweets, such as

soft candies, toffees, taffies, and pastries. If you eat sweets in some occasions, limit them and rinse your mouth with water afterward. Or brush your teeth if you have a chance.

Sugar is harmful to teeth because it can cause tooth decay, which is a result of bacteria in your mouth metabolizing sugar and producing acid. This acid slowly dissolves the enamel on your teeth, creating cavities and holes.

When you drink soda & such cold drinks, the sugars it contains interact with bacteria in your mouth to form acid. This acid attacks your teeth causing teeth decay & cavity. Both regular and sugar-free sodas also contain their own acids, and these attack the teeth too. Erosion begins when the acids in soft drinks encounter the tooth enamel, which is the outermost protective layer on your teeth. Their effect is to reduce the surface hardness of the enamel. While sports drinks and fruit juices can also damage enamel, they stop there.

- Take hard fruits like carrot, apples, guava, nuts etc. and eat them directly by your teeth, after washing them ell with fresh warm water. It gives exercise to your teeth and keep them healthy.

3.11. Skin

The skin is the large organ that covers and protects your body. Your skin has many functions. skin is your first layer of defence against the outside world. Skin can also give important clues to your overall health. The skin provides a barrier to protect the body from invasion by bacteria and other possible environmental hazards that can be dangerous for human health

It works to:

- Hold in fluid and prevent dehydration.
- Help you feel sensations, such as temperature or pain.
- Keep out bacteria, viruses and other causes of infection.
- Stabilize your body temperature.
- Synthesize (create) vitamin D in response to sun exposure.

Skin plays other roles, too. It contains nerve endings that let you feel when an object is too hot or sharp, so you can quickly pull away. Sweat glands and tiny blood vessels in your skin help to control your body temperature.

And cells in your skin turn sunlight into vitamin D, which is important for healthy bones.

Skin can also alert you to a health problem. A red, itchy rash might signal allergies or infections, and a red "butterfly" rash on your face might be a sign of lupus. A yellow tint might indicate liver disease. And dark or unusual moles might be a warning sign of skin cancer. Be on the lookout for unexpected changes to your skin and talk with your doctor if you have concerns.

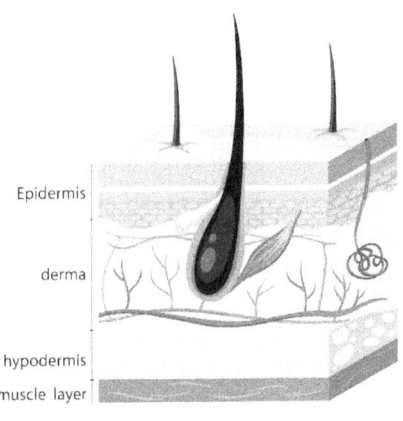

SKIN ANATOMY

Your skin can become too dry if you don't drink enough fluids or spend too much time in sunny or dry conditions. To treat dry skin, use moisturizing creams or lotions, and use warm instead of hot water when you bathe and wash your hands. You can also try using a humidifier to make the air in your home less dry.

The sun can damage your skin as well. Sunlight contains ultraviolet (UV) light that causes sunburn and makes your skin age faster, leading to more wrinkles as you get older. Wear hats and other protective clothing and restrict your time in the sun during the late morning and early afternoon hours, when sunlight is strongest.

Tips for Healthy Skin

Wash up. Bathe in normal or warm — not hot — water; use mild cleansers that don't irritate; and wash gently — don't scrub.

Block sun damage. Avoid intense sun exposure, use sunscreen, and wear protective clothing. Wear sunscreen, sunglasses, and protective clothing when you're outside. Sun exposure can cause wrinkles, age spots, and skin cancer. Avoid tanning beds, which emit harmful UV radiation.

Eat a healthy diet: Eat plenty of fruits, vegetables, lean proteins, and healthy fats.

Avoid dry skin. Drink plenty of water, and use gentle moisturizers, lotions, or creams. Choose the right products, use skin care products formulated for your skin type.

Don't smoke: Smoking can make your skin look older and contribute to wrinkles

Reduce stress. Stress can harm your skin and other body systems. Uncontrolled stress can make your skin more sensitive and trigger acne

Get enough sleep. Sleep helps your body refresh and renew itself. Experts recommend about 9 hours a night for teens and 7-8 hours for adults.

Avoid sharing items: Don't share lip balm, soap, toothbrushes, clothes, or drinks with people who might have any ski disease, cold sores etc.

Check-up. Talk to your doctor/ dermatologist, if you notice any odd changes to your skin, like a rash or mole that changes size or colour.

CHAPTER 4

Prevent some serious diseases to affect you

4.1 Constipation

Lack of timely and proper stool is a symptom of 'constipation'. Constipation is the root cause of all diseases hence eliminating constipation should be the first task for a healthy life.

The biggest reason for constipation is wrong eating habits and food. If we have food with more fibres, we do not take packaged food nor fast foods, take enough green vegetables and salads with sprouted chickpeas and raw onions, seasonal fruits, etc. as a part of our daily diet, then chances of constipation will be zero. Always avoid oily foods and packaged foods to eliminate constipation. In its place take fresh food, salads, nuts & resins, vegetables and fruits, which are rich in fibre and decrease the chance of constipation.

Another reason for constipation is not defecating on time even if there is an urge for it due to workload or negligence. Make it a rule of your life that <u>"if you feel like to go or not to go to toilet for defecation, you must go and if you feel whether to eat or not, you must not eat."</u>

If constipation does not go away due to any reason, then it is advisable to take some Indian or Unani Ayurvedic herbs like Triphala (powder of herbs Harre-Bahera-Amla) - soak a spoon full in water at night and drink it in the morning or take other Unani or Indian Ayurvedic medicines available in the stores in the prescribed quantity at night so that there is stool and constipation does not occur. But these medicines should not become a habit. I firmly believe that constipation will definitely go away with proper daily eating habits of fresh & hot foods cooked in your kitchen taking with enough green vegetable-salads-sprouted grains-fruits etc.

4.2 Heart-attack, strokes and brain haemorrhage

To prevent heart attack, stroke, and brain haemorrhage, you can:

- Maintain a healthy weight: Being overweight or obese increases the risk of heart disease and stroke.
- Improve your lifestyle: The tips mentioned in chapter one can protect us from many diseases including heart-attack & strokes.
- Eat a healthy diet: Eat a diet rich in fruits and vegetables and low in salt. This can help reduce fatty deposits in the arteries and the risk of burst vessels.
- Exercise regularly: Try to get at least 30 minutes of moderate-intensity aerobic activity at least five times a week.

- Manage stress: Try muscle relaxation, breathing techniques, or visualizations.
- Control your blood pressure: High blood pressure is the most potent risk factor for stroke.
- Control your cholesterol and blood sugar levels: Keep these levels in the normal range. Diabetes increases the risk of heart attack.
- Quit smoking: Smoking is a major risk factor for heart disease and stroke.
- Treat heart disease: If you have heart disease, get treatment.

Early warning signs of a stroke include:

- Weakness on one side of the body. A person having a stroke often has muscle weakness on one side. Ask them to raise their arms. If they have one-sided weakness (and didn't have it before), one arm will stay higher while the other will sag and drop downward.
- Numbness of the face. Ask the person to smile. Look for a droop on one or both sides of their face, which is a sign of muscle weakness or paralysis. Strokes often cause a person to lose their ability to speak. They might slur their speech or have trouble choosing the right words
- Unusual and severe headache
- Sudden Vision loss or experiencing double vision
- Numbness and tingling. Sudden loss of balance
- Unsteady walk

- Time is critical, so don't wait to get help! If possible, look at your watch or a clock and remember when symptoms start. Telling a healthcare provider when symptoms started can help the provider know what treatment options are best for you.

4.3 Piles/ haemorrhoids

Piles are the result of swollen veins in the lower anus and rectum. They can cause tissue growths in and around the anus and can lead to significant discomfort. These growths can vary in size and location.

Piles is a very common disease affecting millions of people. As per an estimate it affects about 4.4% of the general population worldwide.

Piles may be caused by too much straining on the toilet, due to prolonged constipation – this is often due to a lack of fibre in a person's diet. Chronic (long-term) diarrhoea can also make you more vulnerable to getting haemorrhoids.

Piles can be prevented by following a healthy lifestyle. Here are some tips to help prevent piles:

- Eat fibre-rich foods: Eat more fruits, vegetables, and whole grains, or take supplements. Fiber helps keep stools soft and easy to pass.
- Practicing Ganesh Kriya and Ashwini Mudra as explained in chapter one.
- Drink plenty of fluids: Drinking water and other fluids helps keep stools soft.

- Exercise regularly: Physical activity helps keep bowels moving.
- Avoid sitting too long on the toilet: Limit the time you spend on the toilet, and don't strain during bowel movements.
- Avoid excessive caffeine and alcohol: Limit caffeinated drinks like tea and coffee, and don't drink too much alcohol.
- Go to the toilet when you need to: Don't delay bowel movements.
- Avoid using too many laxatives or enemas: Using too many can make it hard for your body to regulate bowel movements

4.4, Diabetes

Diabetes is another very common disease. It is caused mainly due to unhealthy lifestyle. If we follow the tips given in chapter one of this book, we can avoid diabetes to a great extent.

As per WHO (https://www.who.int/news-room/fact-sheets/detail/diabetes#:~:text=The%20number%20of%20people%20with,stroke%20and%20lower%20limb%20amputation.)

Key facts

- The number of people with diabetes rose from 108 million in 1980 to 422 million in 2014. Prevalence has been rising more rapidly in low- and middle-income countries than in high-income countries.

- Diabetes is a major cause of blindness, kidney failure, heart attacks, stroke and lower limb amputation.
- Between 2000 and 2019, there was a 3% increase in diabetes mortality rates by age.
- In 2019, diabetes and kidney disease due to diabetes caused an estimated 2 million deaths.
- A healthy diet, regular physical activity, maintaining a normal body weight and avoiding tobacco use are ways to prevent or delay the onset of type 2 diabetes.
- Diabetes can be treated, and its consequences avoided or delayed with diet, physical activity, medication and regular screening and treatment for complications.

Overview

Diabetes is a chronic disease that occurs either when the pancreas does not produce enough insulin or when the body cannot effectively use the insulin it produces. Insulin is a hormone that regulates blood glucose. Hyperglycaemia, also called raised blood glucose or raised blood sugar, is a common effect of uncontrolled diabetes and over time leads to serious damage to many of the body's systems, especially the nerves and blood vessels.

In 2014, 8.5% of adults aged 18 years and older had diabetes. In 2019, diabetes was the direct cause of 1.5 million deaths and 48% of all deaths due to diabetes occurred before the age of 70 years. Another 460 000 kidney disease deaths were caused by diabetes and raised blood glucose causes around 20% of cardiovascular deaths *(1)*.

Between 2000 and 2019, there was a 3% increase in age-standardized mortality rates from diabetes. In lower-middle-income countries, the mortality rate due to diabetes increased 13%.

By contrast, the probability of dying from any one of the four main noncommunicable diseases (cardiovascular diseases, cancer, chronic respiratory diseases or diabetes) between the ages of 30 and 70 decreased by 22% globally between 2000 and 2019.

Symptoms

Symptoms of diabetes may occur suddenly. In type 2 diabetes, the symptoms can be mild and may take many years to be noticed.

Symptoms of diabetes include:

- feeling very thirsty
- needing to urinate more often than usual
- blurred vision
- feeling tired
- losing weight unintentionally

Over time, diabetes can damage blood vessels in the heart, eyes, kidneys and nerves.

People with diabetes have a higher risk of health problems including heart attack, stroke and kidney failure.

Diabetes can cause permanent vision loss by damaging blood vessels in the eyes.

Many people with diabetes develop problems with their feet from nerve damage and poor blood flow. This can cause foot ulcers and may lead to amputation.

Prevention

Lifestyle changes are the best way to prevent or delay the onset of type 2 diabetes.

To help prevent type 2 diabetes and its complications, people should:

- reach and keep a health body weight
- stay physically active with at least 30 minutes of moderate exercise each day
- eat a healthy diet and avoid sugar and saturated fat
- not smoke tobacco.

4.5. Cancer

Cancer is a leading cause of death worldwide. Cancer is a group of diseases that occur when abnormal cells grow and spread uncontrollably in the body. These abnormal cells can form tumours in organs and tissues, or crowd out normal cells in the blood and bone marrow

Cancer is a disease in which some of the body's cells grow uncontrollably and spread to other parts of the body.

Cancer can start almost anywhere in the human body, which is made up of trillions of cells. Normally, human cells grow and multiply (through a process called cell division) to form new cells as the body needs them. When cells grow old or become damaged, they die, and new cells take their place.

Sometimes this orderly process breaks down, and abnormal or damaged cells grow and multiply when they shouldn't. These cells may form tumours, which are lumps of tissue. Tumours can be cancerous or not cancerous (benign).

Cancerous tumours spread into, or invade, nearby tissues and can travel to distant places in the body to form new tumours (a process called metastasis). Cancerous tumours may also be called malignant tumours. Many cancers form solid tumours, but cancers of the blood, such as leukemias, generally do not.

Benign tumours do not spread into, or invade, nearby tissues. When removed, benign tumours usually don't grow back, whereas cancerous tumours sometimes do. Benign tumours can sometimes be quite large, however. Some can cause serious symptoms or be life threatening, such as benign tumours in the brain. (https://www.cancer.gov/about-cancer/understanding/what-is-cancer)

Some risk factors for cancer include:

- Tobacco use: Smoking and using smokeless tobacco can cause cancer. Two out of three deaths from smoking are directly related to smoking.
- Alcohol consumption: Drinking more than one drink a day for women and two drinks a day for men can increase the risk of cancer.

- Obesity: Being overweight or obese can increase the risk of many types of cancer.
- Diet: A low intake of fruits and vegetables can increase the risk of cancer.
- Lack of physical activity: Not getting enough exercise can increase the risk of cancer.
- Air pollution: Air pollution is a risk factor for lung cancer.
- Infections: Some infections, such as human papillomavirus (HPV) and hepatitis, can cause cancer.
- Exposure to radiation: Exposure to ultraviolet (UV) radiation, such as from the sun, can increase the risk of skin cancer.

Prevention

There are many ways to reduce the risk of cancer, including:

- Avoiding tobacco use
- Maintaining a healthy weight
- Have a healthy lifestyle
- Eating a healthy diet
- Exercising regularly
- Limiting alcohol use
- Practicing safe sex
- Getting vaccinated against HPV and hepatitis B
- Reducing exposure to UV radiation
- Getting regular medical care

Early detection of cancer can save your life. Screening tests are important for finding cancer early, when it's most treatable.

CHAPTER 5

Food Items that may be helpful to Keep you Disease Free

The below mentioned food items I have used in my life to be disease free hence I am writing about them, maybe you too find them useful in your life to get protected against many diseases. Include the below food items with great medicinal properties in your daily diet to remain healthy and have improved immunity power and body stamina to stop disease to affect you.

5.1. Indian gooseberry or Amla

Indian gooseberry, or amla, is a fruit rich in vitamin C and often purported to have potential antioxidant and heart-health benefits. I know a person, at the age of about 80, using Amla in his daily diet in the form of "Chatney" (grinded fresh amala mixed with little salt) with lunch & dinner or juice in the morning with breakfast or powdered amala when not available fresh taken with water daily and he is as fit as a youth at the age of 45 having almost no disease. Amla can be taken in many other forms too like pickles, candy or murabba (sweet)

There are numerous Amla benefits and uses as follows: Improves Immunity: Amla benefits include antibacterial & astringent properties which help improve the body's immunity system. Indian Gooseberry also increases white blood cells which help flush out the toxins from the body.

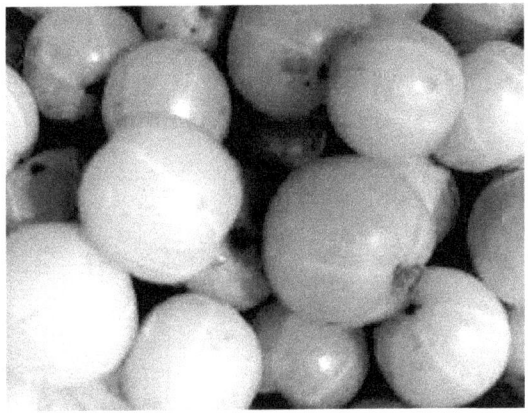

Hair Care: Amla is rich antioxidant & iron content. Indian Gooseberry contains high levels of Vitamin C which helps reduce hair fall. It also strengthens the roots & maintains hair colour. Antibacterial properties of Amla help fight dandruff.

Reduces Stress: Amla is a great stress reliever which helps induce sleep and relieve headaches.

Eye Care: Amla is rich in carotene content which is well known for its powerful effect on vision-related conditions. Formulation made of Indian Gooseberry and Honey helps to improve eyesight, near-sightedness, and cataracts.

Respiratory Health: Amla proves beneficial against respiratory disorders. It helps to reduce cough, tuberculosis, throat infections and flu.

Treats Anaemia: Amla is a rich source of iron, deficiency of which causes anaemia.

Blood Purifier: Amla acts as an active blood purifier when consumed with honey.

Diuretic: Amla is also diuretic in nature. It means that Indian Gooseberry helps increase the volume and frequency of urination which improves the elimination of toxins from the body. Know more on detoxification.

Improve Digestion: Amla is rich in dietary fiber which helps improve the overall digestion process.

Absorbs Calcium: Amla benefits also include absorbing calcium, which is an essential element for teeth, bones & hair.

Anti-aging: Amla reduces the number of free radicals in the body through its antioxidant properties. It helps reduce wrinkles, dark circles and other signs of aging. It also protects the body from radiation. Due to its high vitamin C content, an antioxidant that can help prevent cellular damage, which may help slow our body's natural aging process

Improves Mental Functions: Daily consumption of Amla helps improves nerve health facilitating proper blood flow. It helps to prevent diseases like dementia and Alzheimer's. Indian Gooseberry also helps improve concentration power and memory skills.

Weight Management: Amla is known to boost metabolism which helps reduce body fat. It is recommended to add Amla in one's daily diet.

Skin Care: Amla helps flush out the harmful toxins from the body reducing skin blemishes. The astringent properties of Indian Gooseberry help tighten the pores, giving you clear and healthy skin.

Reduces blood pressure. Indian gooseberry may help reduce high blood pressure levels by acting as a vasodilator, or by widening the blood vessels. High blood pressure is a risk factor for heart disease

5.2. Garlic

I have used garlic in my life very much to control getting cold & cough very often, to improve my immunity, to regulate my blood pressure and have found it very effective. I had taken garlic early in the morning before the breakfast – 3 or 4 cloves grinded with almonds and resins in the mixy. Sometimes I boil it in the milk and drink.

Referring the website on garlic:
https://www.dabur.com/ayurveda/ayurvedic-medicinal-plants/garlic

Hindi Name: **Lashun;** Sanskrit Name: **Rason;** English Name: **Garlic**

Latin Name: **Allium sativum**

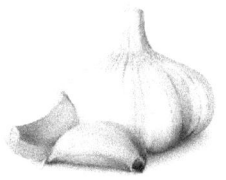

Garlic Benefits and Uses:

Garlic has a very long folk history of use in a wide range of ailments such as ringworm, Candida and vaginitis where its fungicidal, antiseptic, tonic and parasiticidal properties have proved of benefit as recommended by Indian Ayurveda.

1. **Treats Dysentery**

The plant produces inhibitory effects on gram-negative germs of the typhoid-paratyphoid-enteritis group, indeed it possesses outstanding germicidal properties and can keep amoebic dysentery at bay. Garlic benefits also include anticancer activity.

2. **Controls Diabetes**

Benefits of Garlic include reducing glucose metabolism in diabetics, slows the development of arteriosclerosis and lowers the risk of further heart attacks in myocardial infarct patients. Externally, the expressed juice is an excellent antiseptic for treating wounds.

3. **Lowers Cholesterol**

There are two kinds of cholesterol. LDL cholesterol and HDL cholesterol. The former is bad for human health. Garlic is rich in the Ellison compound which effectively prevents LDL cholesterol from oxidizing. All those who have high cholesterol levels should include this herb in their daily diet.

4. Thrombosis

Benefits of Garlic include fighting against thrombosis by reducing platelet aggregation for eye care. Garlic is rich in nutrients like selenium quercetin and vitamin C, all of which help treat infections and swelling.

5. Treats Acne

Half the people in the world suffer from mild to severe forms of acne. Uses of Garlic include treating acne. Garlic may be used, along with other ingredients like honey, cream and turmeric, to treat acne scars and prevent the initial development of acne garlic acts as a cleanser and an antibiotic substance for soothing skin rashes.

6. Heart Health

Garlic protects our heart against cardiovascular problems like heart attacks and atherosclerosis. This cardio protective property can be attributed to various factors. With age, the arteries tend to lose their ability to stretch. Garlic, helps reduce this and may also protect the heart from the damaging effects of free oxygen radicals.

7. Respiratory Problems

Daily use of garlic might reduce the frequency and number of colds. Its antibacterial properties, help in treating throat irritations. Garlic may also reduce the severity of up respiratory tract infections. Its benefits in disorders of the lungs like asthma, difficulty of breathing make it a priceless medicine.

8. **Weight Management**

Many researchers believe that obesity is a state of long-term low-grade inflammation. According to recent research, garlic may help to regulate the formation of fat cells in our body. This may help prevent weight gain.

5.3. Turmeric

(Reference: https://www.healthline.com/nutrition/top-10-evidence-based-health-benefits-of-turmeric#bottom-line)

10 Health Benefits of Turmeric and Curcumin: Many high-quality studies show that turmeric has major benefits for your body and brain. Many of these benefits come from its main active ingredient, curcumin. The spice known as turmeric could be one of the most effective nutritional supplements in existence.

What are turmeric and curcumin? Turmeric is the spice that gives curry its yellow colour. It has been used in India for thousands of years as both a spice and medicinal herb. Research has shown that turmeric contains compounds with medicinal properties.

These compounds are called curcuminoids. The most important one is curcumin, which is the main active ingredient in turmeric.

Here are the top 10 evidence-based health benefits of turmeric and curcumin.

1. Turmeric contains bioactive compounds with medicinal properties: It has powerful anti-inflammatory effects and is a very strong antioxidant. That said, the

curcumin content of turmeric is only around 1-6% by weight. Most studies on this

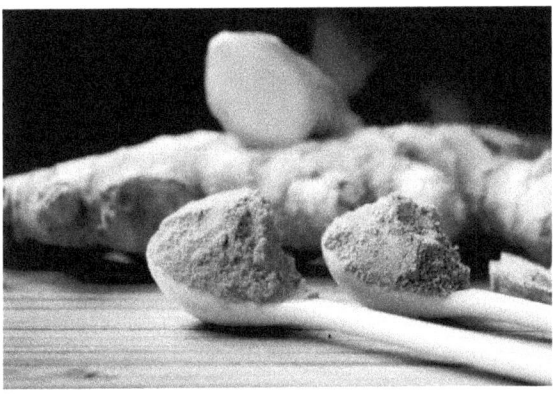

herb use turmeric extracts that contain mostly curcumin itself, with dosages usually exceeding 1 gram (g) per day, which means it would be hard to reach these levels just by using turmeric as a spice. That's why some people choose to use supplements.

In addition, curcumin is poorly absorbed into your bloodstream. In order to experience the full effects of curcumin, its bioavailability (the rate at which your body absorbs a substance) needs to improve.

It helps to consume it with black pepper, which contains piperine. Piperine is a natural substance that enhances the absorption of curcumin by 2,000%. In fact, the best curcumin supplements contain piperine, and this makes them substantially more effective. Curcumin is also fat soluble, which means it breaks down and dissolves in fat or oil. That's why it may be a good idea to take curcumin supplements with a meal that's high in fat.

2. Curcumin is a natural anti-inflammatory compound. Curcumin is a bioactive substance that can help fight inflammation, though very high doses are required to produce medicinal results.

Still, it means it has the potential to fight the inflammation that plays a role in many health conditions and diseases. That's why anything that can help fight chronic inflammation is potentially important in preventing and helping treat these conditions.

3. Turmeric can increase the antioxidant capacity of the body: Oxidative damage is believed to be one of the mechanisms behind aging and many diseases. It involves free radicals, highly reactive molecules with unpaired electrons. Free radicals tend to react with important organic substances, such as fatty acids, proteins, or DNA. Curcumin is a potent antioxidant that can neutralize free radicals due to its chemical structure.

In addition, animal and cellular studies suggest that curcumin may block the action of free radicals and may stimulate the action of other antioxidants. Further clinical studies are needed in humans to confirm these benefits.

4. Curcumin can boost brain-derived neurotrophic factor: Even in adulthood, brain neurons are capable of forming new connections, and in certain areas of the brain, they can multiply and increase in number.

One of the main drivers of this process is brain-derived neurotrophic factor (BDNF), which plays a role in memory and learning, and it can be found in areas of the brain responsible for eating, drinking, and body weight.

Many common brain disorders have been linked to decreased levels of BDNF protein, including depression and Alzheimer's disease.

Both animal and human studies have found that curcumin may increase brain levels of BDNF. By doing this, it may be effective in delaying or even reversing many brain diseases and age-related decreases in brain function. It may also help improve memory and attention, which seems logical given its effects on BDNF levels. However, more studies are needed to confirm this.

5. Curcumin may lower your risk of heart disease: Heart disease is the number one cause of death in the world. Research suggests that curcumin may help protect against many steps in the heart disease process. Specifically, it helps improve the function of the endothelium or the lining of your blood vessels.

Endothelial dysfunction is a major driver of heart disease. This is when your endothelium is unable to regulate blood pressure, blood clotting, and various other factors. Several other studies also suggest that curcumin can lead to improvements in heart health. In addition, curcumin can help reduce inflammation and oxidation (as discussed above), which can play a role in heart disease.

6. Turmeric may help prevent cancer: Many different forms of cancer appear to be affected by curcumin supplements. In fact, curcumin has been studied as a beneficial herb in cancer treatment and has been found to affect cancer growth and development.

Studies have shown that it can: contribute to the death of cancerous cells; reduce angiogenesis (growth of new blood vessels in tumours); reduce metastasis (spread of cancer); There is also evidence that curcumin may prevent cancer from occurring in the first place, especially cancers of the digestive system like colorectal cancer.

7. Curcumin may be useful in treating Alzheimer's disease: Alzheimer's disease is the most common form of dementia and may contribute to up to 70% of dementia cases.

It's known that inflammation and oxidative damage play a role in Alzheimer's disease, and curcumin has been found to have beneficial effects on both. In addition, research suggests that curcumin can help clear the buildup of protein tangles called amyloid plaques that are caused by the disease. That said, whether curcumin can slow or even reverse the progression of Alzheimer's disease in people is currently unknown and needs to be studied.

8. Arthritis patients respond well to curcumin supplements: There are several different types of arthritis, most of which involve inflammation in the joints. In a study on people with osteoarthritis, curcumin appeared to be more effective in relieving pain than a placebo, and research has also found its effect to be similar to that of non-steroidal anti-inflammatory drugs (NSAIDs).

In another study on rheumatoid arthritis, curcumin appeared to have helped reduce disease-related inflammation. That said, more study is needed to understand if curcumin can actually replace such drugs as a treatment for arthritis inflammation pain.

9. Curcumin has benefits against depression: Curcumin has shown some promise in treating mood disorders. Its positive effects on the brain include boosting the brain neurotransmitters serotonin and dopamine, reducing inflammation, and encouraging brain plasticity. This suggests the herb may be an effective antidepressant.

Depression is also linked to reduced levels of BDNF and a shrinking hippocampus, a brain area with a role in learning and memory. Curcumin can help boost BDNF levels, potentially reversing some of these changes.

A 2018 animal study also found that curcumin may help reduce anxiety, though studies on humans are needed to verify this.

10. Curcumin may help delay aging and fight age-related chronic diseases: If curcumin can really help prevent heart disease, cancer, and Alzheimer's, it may have benefits for longevity as well. This suggests that curcumin may have potential as an anti-aging supplement. Given that oxidation and inflammation are believed to play a role in aging, curcumin may have effects that go way beyond just preventing disease.

Frequently asked questions

Is it good to take turmeric every day?

Given turmeric's various beneficial properties to health, it's not a bad idea to take it daily. If you stick to 12 g or less, you are not likely to experience side effects such as diarrhoea, constipation, or vomiting. Learn more about turmeric dosage.

Who shouldn't take turmeric?

People who are pregnant or nursing, people who have gallbladder or kidney problems, those with bleeding disorders, diabetes, or iron deficiency should limit turmeric. If you have any of these conditions, ask your doctor before taking turmeric. Also, ask your doctor if turmeric would interact with any medications you're taking.

Can turmeric burn belly fat?

There is research suggesting that curcumin, the main component of turmeric, might help with reducing belly fat. Learn more: Does turmeric help you lose weight?

The bottom line

Turmeric — and especially its most active compound, curcumin — has many scientifically proven health benefits, such as the potential to improve heart health and prevent Alzheimer's and cancer. It's a potent anti-inflammatory and antioxidant. It may also help improve symptoms of depression and arthritis. While these benefits are possible, they are limited at this time because of curcumin's scarce bioavailability and more research is needed.

Last medically reviewed on November 20, 2023

5.4. Onion

(Reference: https://www.healthline.com/nutrition/onion-benefits)

In my daily salads with lunch and dinner, I take onion and tomato with lemon with a little pinch of rock-salt. I have found it useful to keep me healthy and disease free. As per reference above the 9 Impressive Health Benefits of Onions are

Onions are highly nutritious vegetables that may have several benefits, including improved heart health, better blood sugar regulation, and increased bone density.

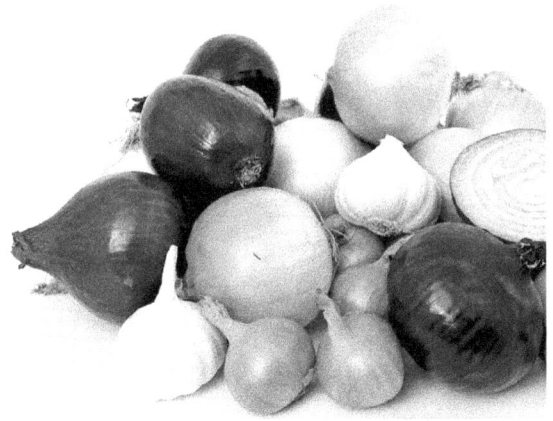

Onions are members of the Allium genus of flowering plants, which also includes garlic, shallots, and leeks. They're delicious, versatile, and relatively cheap, and they boast a wide range of healthy vitamins, minerals, and plant compounds.

The medicinal properties of onions have been recognized for thousands of years. Athletes in ancient Greece supposedly used onions to purify their blood, while medieval and traditional doctors prescribed them to help treat headaches, heart disease, and mouth sores.

Read on to discover 9 health benefits of onions.

1. Packed with nutrients: Onions are nutrient-dense, meaning they're low in calories but high in vitamins, fibre, and minerals.

One medium onion (110 grams [g]) contains: Calories: 44; Protein: 1.2 g; Carbs: 10.3 g; Sugar: 4.7 g; Fiber: 1.9 g; Fat: 0.1 g; Potassium: 3.4% of Daily Value (DV); Vitamin C: 9% of the DV

Onions are high in vitamin C, which may help regulate your immune health, collagen production, and iron absorption. It's also a powerful antioxidant that could help protect your cells from unstable, damaging molecules called free radicals.

Onions are rich in B vitamins, including folate and vitamin B6. These play key roles in metabolism, red blood cell production, and nerve function.

Lastly, onions are a good source of potassium, a mineral that may help with: cellular function; fluid balance; nerve transmission; kidney function; muscle contraction; adding onions to your diet is a great way to increase your potassium intake.

2. May benefit heart health: Onions contain antioxidants and compounds that may reduce your risk of heart disease by fighting inflammation and lowering triglyceride and cholesterol levels. They contain a large

amount of quercetin, a flavonoid antioxidant and anti-inflammatory that may help lower high blood pressure.

A small 2015 study in 70 people with overweight and hypertension suggests that a daily dose of 162 mg of quercetin-rich onion extract may significantly reduce systolic blood pressure by 3.6 millimetres of mercury.

Also, a small 2014 study in 54 females with polycystic ovary syndrome found that consuming 80–120 g of raw red onions per day for 8 weeks lowered total and LDL (bad) cholesterol levels. However, more research is needed.

3. Loaded with antioxidants: Antioxidants are compounds that inhibit oxidation, a process that may lead to cellular damage and contribute to diseases such as cancer, diabetes, and heart disease.

Onions are an excellent source of antioxidants and contain at least 17 types of flavonoids. Red onions, in particular, contain anthocyanins, plant pigments in the flavonoid family that give red onions their deep colour. These may protect against diabetes and certain types of cancer.

In a 2016 study involving 43,880 males, researchers found that habitual anthocyanin intakes up to 613 mg were correlated with a 14% lower risk of nonfatal heart attacks.

Similarly, the authors of a 2019 review concluded that consuming more anthocyanin-rich foods was associated with a lower risk of heart disease and of death from heart disease.

4. Contain anticancer compounds: Allium vegetables such as onions and garlic may lower your risk of developing certain types of cancer, including stomach and colorectal cancers.

In a 2015 review of 26 studies, researchers concluded that people who consumed the most allium vegetables were 22% less likely to receive a diagnosis of stomach cancer than those who consumed the least.

And in a 2014 review of 16 studies involving a total of 13,333 people, researchers suggested that people with the greatest onion intake had a 15% lower risk of colorectal cancer than those with the lowest intake.

Test-tube studies suggest that onionin A, a sulphur-containing compound in onions, may help decrease tumour development and slow the spread of ovarian cancer. Onions also contain fisetin and quercetin, which are flavonoid antioxidants that may inhibit tumour growth.

5. Help regulate blood sugar: Eating onions may help regulate blood sugar levels, which is significant for people with diabetes or prediabetes.

A small 2010 study in 84 people with type 1 or type 2 diabetes found that eating 100 g of raw red onion significantly reduced fasting blood sugar levels after 4 hours.

A 2020 study showed that rats with diabetes who ate food containing 5% dried onion powder for 8 weeks had decreased fasting blood sugar levels and lower triglyceride and cholesterol levels than a control group.

Quercetin has also been shown to help regulate whole-body blood sugar balance by interacting with cells in the: small intestine; pancreas; skeletal muscle; fat tissue; liver.

6. May boost bone density: Dairy gets much of the credit for boosting bone health, but other foods, including onions, may also help support strong bones.

A small 2016 study in 24 middle-aged and postmenopausal females found that those who consumed 100 millilitres of onion juice daily for 8 weeks had improved bone mineral density and antioxidant activity compared to a control group.

Also, a 2009 study in 507 perimenopausal and postmenopausal females found that those who ate onions at least once per day had a 5% greater overall bone density than those who ate onions once per month or less often.

Onions may help reduce oxidative stress, boost antioxidant levels, and decrease bone loss. This may help prevent osteoporosis and improve bone density.

7. Have antibacterial properties: Onions may help fight potentially dangerous bacteria such as: Escherichia coli (E. coli); Pseudomonas aeruginosa; Staphylococcus aureus (S. aureus); Bacillus cereus

A 2010 test-tube study suggests that onion extract might inhibit the growth of Vibrio cholerae, a type of bacteria that is a major public health concern in some parts of the world. Quercetin extracted from onions may also reduce bacteria growth.

One review suggests that it could inhibit the growth of several strains of bacteria, including Helicobacter pylori, a type of bacteria associated with stomach ulcers and certain digestive cancers. Another test-tube study found that quercetin damaged the cell walls and membranes of E. coli and S. aureus.

8. May boost digestive health: Onions are a rich source of fibre and prebiotics, which are necessary for optimal gut health. Prebiotics are nondigestible types of fibre that are broken down by beneficial gut bacteria. Gut bacteria feed on prebiotics and create short-chain fatty acids, which may help strengthen gut health; boost immunity; reduce inflammation; enhance digestion. Consuming prebiotic foods may also help increase probiotics, such as Lactobacillus and Bifidobacterium strains, which benefit digestive health.

Onions are rich in the prebiotics inulin and fructooligosaccharides, which may help increase the number of friendly bacteria in your gut and improve immune function.

9. Easy to add to your diet: Onions are a fresh and versatile staple in kitchens around the world. They can be cooked, fried, eaten raw, and more. To incorporate onions into your diet, you can try: using them in soups such as French onion soup; using them in dips and spreads such as guacamole, salsa, and ranch; adding them to egg dishes such as omelettes, frittatas, and quiches; making cooked toppings, such as caramelized onions, to top meat or tofu or add to savory baked goods; using them raw as a topping for tacos, fajitas, and other

Mexican dishes and savory baked goods; adding them to salads, such as a chickpea, chopped onion, and red pepper salad; using them in stir-fries, pasta sauces, or curries

Takeaway

Onions are nutrient-packed vegetables that contain powerful compounds that may help decrease your risk of heart disease and certain cancers. They have antibacterial properties and promote digestive health, which may improve immune function. What's more, they're versatile and can be used to heighten the flavour of any dish.

5.5. Dates

(Reference: https://www.healthline.com/nutrition/benefits-of-dates)

I am used to take dates, with walnuts and almonds in my daily breakfast with fruits, which keeps me free from many disease and keeps me healthy. As per above reference the 8 Proven Health Benefits of Dates are:

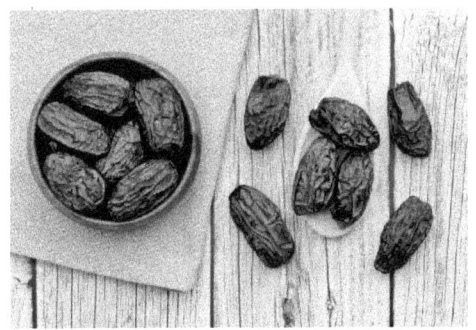

Dates are high in fibre and antioxidants. Their nutritional benefits may support brain health and prevent disease.

Dates are the fruit of the date palm tree, which is grown in many tropical regions of the world. Dates have become quite popular in recent years.

Almost all dates sold in Western countries are dried.

You can tell whether or not dates are dried based on their appearance. Wrinkled skin indicates they are dried, whereas smooth skin indicates freshness.

Depending on the variety, fresh dates are fairly small in size and range in colour from bright red to bright yellow. Commonly consumed varieties include Medjool and Deglet Noor dates.

Dates are chewy with a sweet flavour. They are also high in some important nutrients and have a variety of advantages and uses.

This article will discuss 8 health benefits of eating dates and how to incorporate them into your diet.

1. Very nutritious

Dates have an excellent nutrition profile: Since they're dried, their calorie content is higher than most fresh fruit. The calorie content of dates is similar to that of other dried fruits, such as raisins and figs.

Most of the calories in dates come from carbs. The rest are from a very small amount of protein. Despite their calories, dates contain some important vitamins and minerals in addition to a significant amount of fibre.

A 3.5-ounce (100-gram) serving of Medjool dates provides the following nutrients: **Calories:** 277; **Carbs:** 75 grams; **Fiber:** 7 grams; **Protein:** 2 grams; **Potassium:** 15% DV; **Magnesium**: 13% DV; **Copper:** 40% DV; **Manganese:** 13% DV; **Iron:** 5% DV; **Vitamin B6:** 15% DV

Dates are also high in antioxidants, which may contribute to many of their health benefits (4Trusted Source).

Summary: Dates contain several vitamins and minerals, in addition to fibre and antioxidants. However, they are high in calories since they are dried fruit.

2. High in fibre: Getting enough fibre is important for your overall health. With almost 7 grams of fibre in a 3.5-ounce serving, including dates in your diet is a great way to increase your fibre intake.

Fiber can benefit your digestive health by preventing constipation. It promotes regular bowel movements by contributing to the formation of stool.

In one study, 21 people who consumed 7 dates per day for 21 days experienced improvements in stool frequency and had a significant increase in bowel movements compared to when they did not eat dates.

Furthermore, the fibre in dates may be beneficial for blood sugar control. Fiber slows digestion and may help prevent blood sugar levels from spiking too high after eating.

For this reason, dates have a low glycemic index (GI), which measures how quickly your blood sugar rises after eating a certain food .

Summary: Dates are high in fibre, which may be beneficial for preventing constipation and controlling blood sugar.

3. High in disease-fighting antioxidants: Dates provide various antioxidants that have a number of health benefits, including a reduced risk of several diseases.

Antioxidants protect your cells from free radicals, which are unstable molecules that may cause harmful reactions in your body and lead to disease. Compared to similar types of fruit, such as figs and dried plums, dates appear to have the highest antioxidant content (10Trusted Source).

Here's an overview of the three most potent antioxidants in dates:

- **Flavonoids:** Flavonoids are powerful antioxidants that may help reduce inflammation and have been studied for their potential to reduce the risk of diabetes, Alzheimer's disease, and certain types of cancer.
- **Carotenoids:** Carotenoids are proven to promote heart health and may also reduce the risk of eye-related disorders, such as macular degeneration.
- **Phenolic acid:** Known for their anti-inflammatory properties, phenolic acids may help lower the risk of cancer and heart disease.

Summary: Dates contain several types of antioxidants that may help prevent the development of certain chronic illnesses, such as heart disease, cancer, Alzheimer's, and diabetes.

4. May promote brain health: Eating dates may help improve brain function.

Laboratory studies have found dates to be helpful for lowering inflammatory markers, such as interleukin 6 (IL-6), in the brain. High levels of IL-6 are associated with a higher risk of neurodegenerative diseases like Alzheimer's.

Additionally, other studies including animal studies have shown dates to be helpful for reducing the activity of amyloid beta proteins, which can form plaques in the brain.

When plaques accumulate in the brain, they may disturb communication between brain cells, which can ultimately lead to brain cell death and Alzheimer's disease.

One animal study found that mice fed food mixed with dates had significantly better memory and learning ability, as well as less anxiety-related behaviours, compared to those that did not eat them.

The potential brain-boosting properties of dates have been attributed to their content of antioxidants known to reduce inflammation, including flavonoids. However, more human studies are needed to confirm the role of dates in brain health.

Summary: Dates may be helpful for lowering inflammation and preventing plaques from forming in the brain, which may be important for preventing Alzheimer's disease.

5. May promote natural labor: Dates have been studied for their potential to promote and ease late-term labor in pregnant people.

Eating these fruits throughout the last few weeks of pregnancy may promote cervical dilation and lower the need for induced labor. They may also be helpful in reducing labor time.

An older meta-analysis from 2011 looking at studies where pregnant people took dates prior to their due date found those who ate dates were in labor for less time than those who did not eat them, but also notes that the link between eating dates and a faster delivery needs to be researched further .

A 2017 study of 154 pregnant people found that those who ate dates were much less likely to be induced compared to those who did not.

A third study found similar results in 91 pregnant people who consumed 70–76 grams of dates daily starting the 37th week of pregnancy. They were in active labor for an average of 4 fewer hours than those who did not eat dates.

Although eating dates appears to help promote labor and reduce labor duration, more research is needed to confirm these effects.

The role dates may have in pregnancy is likely due to compounds that bind to oxytocin receptors and appear to mimic the effects of oxytocin in the body. Oxytocin is a hormone that causes labor contractions during childbirth.

Additionally, dates contain tannins, which are compounds that have been shown to help facilitate contractions. They are also a good source of natural sugar and calories, which are necessary to maintain energy levels during labor.

Summary: Dates may promote and ease natural labor for pregnant people when consumed during the last few weeks of pregnancy.

6. Natural sweetener: Dates are a source of fructose, which is a natural type of sugar found in fruit.

For this reason, dates are very sweet and also have a subtle caramel-like taste. They make a great healthy substitute for white sugar in recipes due to the nutrients, fibre, and antioxidants that they provide.

The best way to substitute dates for white sugar is to make date paste, as in this recipe. It is made by mixing dates with water in a blender. A rule of thumb is to replace sugar with date paste at a 1:1 ratio.

For example, if the recipe calls for 1 cup of sugar, you'll replace it with 1 cup of date paste. It is important to note that although dates are high in fibre and nutrients, they are still fairly high in calories and best consumed in moderation.

Summary: Dates are a healthy substitute for white sugar in recipes due to their sweet taste, nutrients, fibre and antioxidants.

7. Other potential health benefits

People claim dates have a few other health benefits that have not yet been extensively studied.

- **Bone health:** Dates contain several minerals, including phosphorus, calcium, and magnesium. All of these have been studied for their potential to prevent bone-related conditions like osteoporosis.
- **Blood sugar control:** Dates have the potential to help with blood sugar regulation due to their low glycemic index, fibre, and antioxidants. Thus, eating them may support diabetes management.

Although these potential health benefits are promising, more human studies are needed before conclusions can be made.

Summary: Some claim dates promote bone health and aid in blood sugar control, but these effects have not been studied sufficiently.

8. Easy to add to your diet: Dates are incredibly versatile and make a delicious snack. They are often paired with other foods, such as almonds, nut butter, or soft cheese.

Dates are also very sticky, which makes them useful as a binder in baked goods, such as cookies and bars. You can also combine dates with nuts and seeds to make healthy snack bars or energy balls, as in this recipe.

What's more, you can use dates to sweeten up sauces, such as salad dressings and marinades, or blend them into smoothies and oatmeal.

It is important to note that dates are high in calories and their sweet taste makes them easy to overeat. For this reason, they are best consumed in moderation.

Summary: There are many different ways to eat dates. They are commonly eaten plain but can also be incorporated into other popular dishes.

The bottom line

Dates are a healthy fruit to include in your diet. They are high in several nutrients, fibre, and antioxidants, all of which may provide health benefits ranging from improved digestion to a reduced risk of disease.

There are several ways to add dates to your diet. One popular way to eat them is as a natural sweetener in various dishes. They also make a great snack. It's easiest to find dates in their dried form, though these are higher in calories than fresh fruit, so it is important to eat them in moderation.

Dates are definitely worth adding to your diet, as they are both nutritious and delicious.

5.6. Raisins

(https://naturalfoodseries.org/11-benefits-raisins/)

11 Impressive Health Benefits of Raisins as per reference above:

By Michael Jessimy / April 28, 2024

Raisins amazing health benefits includes treating anaemia, preventing cancer, promoting proper digestion, combating hair loss, treating skin diseases, treating joint pains, regulating body pH level, relieving fever, support eye health, boosting energy level, supporting dental health, and curing insomnia.

What are Raisins?

Raisins are packed with nature's gifts including all essential minerals, vitamins and antioxidants. Raisins have a phytochemical known as resveratrol, best known for its cholesterol lowering and anti-cancer qualities.

It serves as a nutritious alternative to many of today's chemically processed foods such as chips and crisps. Although they are delicious enough to eat alone, they are a regular component of hundreds of nutritious salads and foods. The popular carrot raisin salad offers a wonderful combination of both crunchy and sweet Flavors. It's easily accessible and available in all local super-markets in large and small containers. Make sure you purchase good quality raisins that are packaged properly.

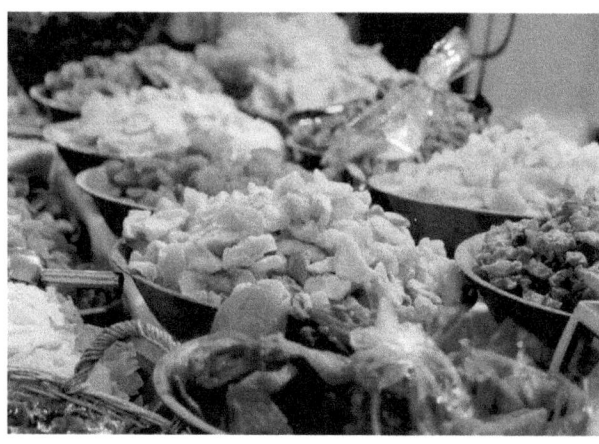

There are dozens of benefits of consuming raisins. Here are a few of the conditions that can be successfully relieved by consuming raisins.

11 Impressive Health Benefits of Raisins

1. Anaemia

Since, it's packed with iron, copper and B complex vitamins; they are a valuable addition to your daily diet. You can steer clear of anaemia or iron deficiency by regularly consuming raisins.

2. Cancer

High levels of polyphenolic antioxidants, known as catechins, hunt for the free radicals that lead to the occurrence of tumors, particularly colon cancer. Including raisins in your diet is a great way to prevent many forms of cancers.

3. Poor Digestion

Raisins are particularly known for containing a rich content of fiber. Hence, they serve as a great remedy to treat chronic constipation. If you want to regularize your bowel movements, use raisins regularly to keep your gastrointestinal tract healthy.

4. Acidity

There are many essential minerals such as magnesium and potassium present in raisins. These are especially helpful in reducing acidity. Moreover, they also relieve many metabolic conditions that lead to blood toxicity.

Hence, they are an effective treatment against many health conditions.

Consuming it is a great way to combat hair loss, skin diseases and joint pain. Raisins help in regulating the body's pH level to prevent acidity and its side effects.

5. Fever

Since they are rich in phenolic phytochemicals, they are great antibacterial and antioxidant agents. Raisins are helpful in relieving bacterial infections or fever caused by viruses.

6. Poor Eye Health

It also include many polyphenolic phytonutrients that are great for ocular health. Because they guard our eyes from many damages caused by free radicals, we can prevent several eye diseases such as macular degeneration and cataracts by regularly consuming raisins.

They are also good sources of vitamin A and beta carotene to improve eyesight for maintaining good eye health.

7. Low Energy

If you feel low, eat a handful of raisins to boost your spirits. They are packed with carbs, especially natural sugars including glucose and fructose. This is why raisins are always handy when you need a quick boost of energy. They also help in good absorption of all essential nutrients including proteins in the body.

It is not surprising to know that many athletes and body builders eat plenty of raisins to elevate their energy levels.

8. Bad Dental Health

Another great benefit of raisins is that it contains a phytochemical called oleanolic acid that offers incredible protection against all kinds of dental problems. If you suffer from cavities, tooth decay or brittle teeth; raisins will prevent any bacterial growth in your mouth. Moreover, raisins are also rich in calcium to protect tooth enamel.

9. Hypertension

If you frequently experience high blood pressure, eat a handful of raisins to give regulate your blood flow. Since they contain many antioxidants along with iron, potassium and B-complex vitamins; It's helpful in reducing the stiffness of blood vessels. This greatly helps in relieving and lowering hypertension. The absence of sodium makes it a great snack during hunger pangs.

10. Cures Insomnia

They are also recommended as a beneficial treatment to help sleep disorders. It's guaranteed to fix a distorted sleep pattern.

11. Poor Bone Health

As mentioned above, raisins also contain good amounts of calcium. This is important to strengthen bones and relieve joint pain. Raisins are also great sources of a micronutrient, boron. Our body needs it in small quantities for efficient calcium absorption and bone formation.

It's also beneficial in preventing menopause induced osteoporosis and supports good bone health.

More Health Benefits of Raisin

There are many other benefits of raisins that do a lot more to help us lead a healthier life. It is often recommended to consume for relieving constipating, lifting energy levels and to improve the quality of our hair and nails.

The rich fibre content helps keep us full for a longer time. It is a great snack if you want to avoid unhealthy food choices. They are also beneficial for weight watchers who want to include natural sugars into their daily diet without increasing their cholesterol levels.

Nutritional Value of Raisin

It greatly helps to eat raisins every day. They also serve as a great laxative owing to its impressive fiber content. Moreover, raisins also keep the bowel movement regular and flush all waste products and toxins out of our system.

They are loaded with all essential nutrients to guarantee exceptionally healthy hair and skin. They also contain vitamin C that helps in maintaining the follicle's connective tissue or more commonly known as collagen. Hence, people who are experiencing hair loss are recommended to consume raisins. Moreover, the vitamin E present in raisins fortifies all the cell membranes in our body to prevent any damage due to free radicals.

Like many dried fruits, they are used for getting a quick energy boost. Raisins are high in calories. Every 100 grams serving offers 249 calories. They offer incredible benefits to maintain good health and to support our immunity.

Anyone who is looking to substitute his unhealthy snacks with naturally sweet foods should definitely include raisins in his diet. They are a healthy way to lose weight since raisins serve as a healthy option to replace unhealthy sweets.

5,7, Walnuts

(https://www.healthline.com/nutrition/benefits-of-walnuts)

As per above reference and on the basis of my personal experiences in daily life by using in the breakfast the 13 Proven Health Benefits of Walnuts are:

Walnuts are a healthy nut chock-full of essential nutrients such as omega-3 fatty acids and antioxidants. They're also easy to incorporate into your diet.

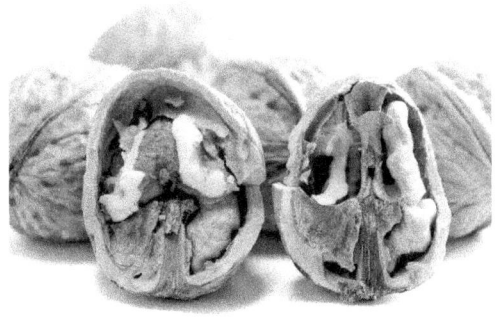

To say that walnuts are a nutritious food is a bit of an understatement.

Walnuts provide healthy fats, fibre, vitamins, and minerals — and that's just the beginning of how they may support your health.

In fact, there's so much interest in this one nut that scientists and industry experts have gathered annually for the past 50 years at the University of California, Davis, for a walnut conference to discuss the latest walnut health research.

The most common variety of walnut is the English walnut (*Juglans regia*), which is also the most studied type.

Here are 13 science-based health benefits of walnuts.

Benefits of walnuts

1. Rich in antioxidants

Walnuts have greater antioxidant activity than any other common nut.

This activity comes from vitamin E, melatonin, and plant compounds called polyphenols, which are found in particularly large amounts in the papery skin of walnuts.

A 2022 study in healthy adults over age 60 showed that eating a walnut-rich meal reduced the participants' levels of LDL (bad) cholesterol.

If LDL cholesterol builds up in your arteries, it can cause atherosclerosis.

Summary: Walnuts are an excellent source of antioxidants that can help lower your LDL (bad) cholesterol level.

2. Super plant source of omega-3s

Walnuts are significantly higher in omega-3 fatty acids than any other nut, providing 2.5 grams (g) per 1-ounce (oz) serving.

Omega-3 fats from plants, including walnuts, is called alpha-linolenic acid (ALA). It's an essential fat, which means you have to get it from your diet.

According to the Institute of Medicine, an adequate intake of ALA is 1.6 g per day for men and 1.1 g per day for women. A single serving of walnuts meets this guideline.

Studies suggest that increased dietary levels of ALA may lower the risk of cardiovascular conditions such as heart disease and arrhythmia.

Summary: Walnuts are a good source of the plant form of omega-3 fat, which may help reduce the risk of cardiovascular diseases and conditions.

3. May decrease inflammation

Inflammation, which can be caused by oxidative stress, is the root of many diseases, including: heart disease' type 2 diabetes; Alzheimer's disease; cancer

The polyphenols in walnuts can help fight oxidative stress and inflammation.

A subgroup of polyphenols called ellagitannins may be especially involved.

Beneficial bacteria in your gut convert ellagitannins to compounds called urolithins, which have been found to protect against inflammation.

ALA, omega-3 fats, magnesium, and the amino acid arginine — all of which are found in walnuts — may also decrease inflammation.

Summary: Several plant compounds and nutrients in walnuts may help decrease inflammation, which is a key culprit in many chronic conditions.

4. Promote a healthy gut

Studies suggest that if your gut is rich in health-promoting bacteria and other microbes (your gut microbiota), you're more likely to have a healthy gut and good overall health.

An unhealthy composition of gut microbiota can contribute to inflammation and disease in your gut and elsewhere in your body, increasing your risk of obesity, heart disease, and cancer.

What you eat can significantly influence the makeup of your microbiota. Eating walnuts may be one way to support the health of your microbiota and your gut.

In a 2018 study, 194 healthy adults ate 1.5 oz (43 g) of walnuts every day for 8 weeks. At the end, they showed an increase in beneficial bacteria compared to a period of not eating walnuts.

This included an increase in bacteria that produce butyrate, a fat that nourishes your gut and promotes gut health.

Summary: Eating walnuts nourishes both you and the beneficial bacteria that live in your gut. This promotes gut health and may help reduce the risk of obesity, heart disease, and cancer.

5. May reduce risk of some cancers

Animal and a few human studies suggest that eating walnuts may reduce your risk of certain cancers, including breast, prostate, and colorectal cancer.

As noted earlier, walnuts are rich in polyphenols called ellagitannins. Certain gut microbes can convert these to compounds called urolithins.

Urolithins can have anti-inflammatory properties in your gut, which may be one way that eating walnuts helps protect against colorectal cancer. These anti-inflammatory actions could also help protect against other cancers.

What's more, urolithins have hormone-like properties that enable them to block hormone receptors in your body. This may help reduce your risk of hormone-related cancers, especially breast and prostate cancers.

But more human studies are needed to determine the effects of eating walnuts on the risk of these and other cancers.

Summary: The polyphenols in walnuts may reduce your risk of certain cancers, including breast, prostate, and colorectal cancers. However, more human studies are needed to learn more about this.

6. Support weight management

Walnuts are calorie-dense, but a small 2016 study suggests that your body absorbs 21% less energy from them than would be expected based on their nutrients.

What's more, eating walnuts may help regulate your appetite.

A well-controlled study in 10 people with obesity found that drinking a smoothie made with about 1.75 oz (48 g) of walnuts once per day for 5 days decreased the participants' appetite and hunger. This was in comparison to a placebo drink equal in calories and nutrients.

Additionally, after 5 days of consuming the walnut smoothies, brain scans showed that the participants had increased activation in a region of the brain that helped them resist highly tempting food cues, such as cake and french fries.

Even though larger and longer-term studies are needed, this provides some initial insight into how walnuts may help regulate appetite and weight.

Summary: Though walnuts are calorie-dense, you may not absorb all the calories they contain. Additionally, they may help regulate your appetite.

7. May help manage and lower your risk for type 2 diabetes

Observational studies suggest that one reason walnuts are linked to a lower risk of type 2 diabetes is that they help manage weight.

Excess weight increases your risk of high blood sugar and diabetes.

Eating walnuts may help regulate blood sugar by mechanisms beyond their influence on weight management.

In a small 2016 study, 100 people with type 2 diabetes consumed 1 tablespoon of cold-pressed walnut oil per day for 3 months while continuing their usual diabetes medication and balanced diet.

This resulted in an 8% decrease in fasting blood sugar.

Additionally, the walnut oil users had about an 8% decrease in haemoglobin A1C (3-month average blood sugar).

The control group showed no improvement in A1C or fasting blood sugar. Neither group had a change in their weight.

Some other research also suggests that supplementing your diet with walnuts could lead to a modest improvement in blood glucose levels.

However, it's important to keep in mind that consuming walnut oil is not the same as eating whole walnuts.

Summary: Consuming walnut oil and walnuts may help manage type 2 diabetes and reduce your risk of the disease by helping to regulate your weight. Walnuts might have more direct effects on blood sugar regulation as well.

8. May help lower blood pressure

High blood pressure is a major risk factor for heart disease and stroke.

A small 2019 study suggests that eating walnuts may help lower blood pressure, including in people with high blood pressure.

Additionally, the authors of a 2019 research review examined the effects of a Mediterranean diet, which often involves consumption of walnuts and other nuts. They concluded that following the Mediterranean diet may help lower blood pressure in some people.

This suggests that nuts may slightly improve the blood pressure benefits of a heart-healthy diet. Even small differences in blood pressure are thought to have a big impact on your risk of heart disease.

Summary: Some studies suggest that eating nuts, including walnuts, daily as part of a heart-healthy diet may help improve blood pressure.

9. Support healthy aging

As you age, good physical functioning is essential for maintaining your mobility and independence.

One thing that may help you maintain your physical abilities is healthy eating habits.

In an observational study involving more than 50,000 women over 18 years, scientists found that those with the healthiest diets had a 13% lower risk of physical impairment.

Walnuts were among the foods that made the strongest contribution to a healthy diet.

Though relatively high in calories, walnuts are packed with essential vitamins, minerals, fiber, fats, and plant compounds that may help support good physical functioning as you age.

Summary: A healthy diet that includes walnuts may help preserve physical function, such as walking and self-care abilities, as you age.

10. Support good brain function

It may be just a coincidence that the shell of a walnut looks like a tiny brain, but research suggests that this nut may indeed be good for your mind.

Animal and human studies suggest that the nutrients and antioxidants in walnuts may help reduce oxidative stress and inflammation by reducing free radicals.

A 2016 study in mice suggests that walnut extract may improve symptoms of Parkinson's disease (PD).

Additionally, a 2019 study in humans found that people with depression showed improvement in symptoms if nuts, including walnuts, were a part of their diet.

Studies in mice have linked eating walnuts to better brain function, including improvements in memory, learning skills, motor development, and anxiety-related behaviour.

Though these results are encouraging, more studies on the effects of walnuts on brain function in humans are needed before researchers can draw firm conclusions.

Summary: Walnuts contain nutrients that may help protect your brain from damaging inflammation and support good brain function as you age.

11. Support reproductive health in people with sperm

Typical Western diets — high in processed foods, sugar, and refined grains — have been linked to reduced sperm function.

Eating walnuts may help support sperm health and male fertility.

In a 2012 study involving 117 healthy young men, participants who ate 2.5 oz (75 g) of walnuts per day for 3 months as part of a Western-style diet had improved sperm shape, vitality and motility compared to those who did not eat nuts.

Animal research suggests that eating walnuts may help protect sperm by reducing oxidative damage in their membranes.

Further studies are needed to learn more about these benefits. But if you have concerns about fertility and sperm function, eating walnuts is a simple thing to try.

Summary: Eating walnuts regularly may help counteract potentially harmful effects of less-than-ideal eating habits on sperm health.

12. Improve blood fat levels

Elevated levels of LDL (bad) cholesterol and triglycerides have long been linked to an increased heart disease risk.

Regularly eating walnuts has been consistently shown to decrease cholesterol levels.

In a small 2017 study in healthy adults, eating 1.5 oz (43 g) of walnuts daily for 8 weeks produced a 5% decrease in total cholesterol, LDL cholesterol, and triglycerides compared to not eating walnuts.

The walnut eaters also had nearly a 6% decrease in apolipoprotein B, which is an indicator of how many LDL particles are in your blood. Elevated apolipoprotein B is a major risk factor for heart disease.

Summary: A daily 1.5-oz (43-g) serving of walnuts may help lower cholesterol and triglyceride levels, which contribute to heart disease risk.

13. Widely available and easy to add to your diet

You can find walnuts in any grocery store. Check for raw walnuts in the baking aisle, roasted walnuts in the nut aisle, and cold-pressed walnut oil in the specialty oils section.

It's helpful to understand how to convert the serving sizes used in studies so that you know how your portion sizes compare.

The following servings are essentially equivalent, providing about 190 calories each: 1 oz shelled walnuts = 28 g = 1/4 cup = 12–14 halves = 1 small handful. Though it's simplest to eat walnuts one by one as a snack, there are plenty of tasty ways to use them in dishes.

Summary: Walnuts are easy to add to your diet since they're widely available in stores and a great addition to countless dishes. Just be wary of any nut allergies.

Frequently asked questions

What are the health benefits of walnuts?

Walnuts have numerous health benefits. For example, they:

- are rich in antioxidants and can reduce LDL (bad) cholesterol
- are significantly higher in omega-3s than any other nut
- may decrease inflammation
- can help promote a healthy gut
- may reduce risk of some cancers
- may help regular appetite and weight
- may help manage and lower your risk for type 2 diabetes
- may help lower your blood pressure
- can benefit brain health
- may improve sperm health and male fertility
- are an excellent source of healthy fats, vitamins, and minerals

How many walnuts should you eat in a day?

A 2021 article the effect of walnut consumption found that consuming 30–60 grams of walnuts daily is beneficial for heart health. 30–60 grams is the same as 1–2 ounces or a 1/4–1/2 cup of walnuts.

Is it safe to eat walnuts every day?

Yes, daily consumption of walnuts is safe. A 2017 study examined the effects of a eating 43 grams (1.5 ounces) of walnuts every day for 8 weeks and found that it led to positive health effects.

Are walnuts better for you than almonds?

Walnuts and almonds both provide health benefits. Determining which one is better for you depends on your health goals.

If you want to target brain health, walnuts are your go-to. But if you're looking to boost your intake of nutrients such as vitamin E, phosphorus, and magnesium, almonds might be the better choice.

The bottom line

Walnuts are an exceptionally nutritious nut. They have greater antioxidant activity and significantly more healthy omega-3 fatty acids than any other common nut.

This rich nutrient profile contributes to the many health benefits associated with walnuts, such as reduced inflammation and improved heart disease risk factors.

Scientists are still uncovering the many ways that walnuts' fiber and plant compounds, including polyphenols, may interact with your gut microbiota and contribute to your health.

It's likely that you'll hear more about walnuts in the years to come as more researchers study their potential health benefits.

Still, there are plenty of reasons to try a walnut-enriched diet.

5.8. Almonds

(https://www.healthline.com/nutrition/9-proven-benefits-of-almonds)

Evidence-Based Health Benefits of Almonds

Almonds are high in antioxidants, vitamin E, protein, and fiber. Almonds may have health benefits, including supporting heart health and reducing blood pressure, among others.

Almonds are among the world's most popular tree nuts.

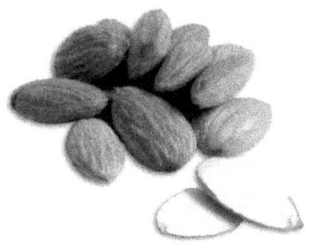

They are highly nutritious and rich in healthy fats, antioxidants, vitamins, and minerals.

Here are 9 health benefits of almonds.

1. Almonds deliver a massive amount of nutrients

Almonds are the edible seeds of *Prunus dulcis*, more commonly called the almond tree.

They are native to the Middle East, but the United States is now the world's largest producer.

The almonds you can buy in stores usually have the shell removed, revealing the edible nut inside. They are sold either raw or roasted.

They are also used to produce products like almond milk, oil, butter, flour, paste, or marzipan.

Almonds boast an impressive nutrient profile. A 1-ounce (oz), or 28-gram (g), serving of almonds contains: **Fiber:** 3.5 g; **Protein:** 6 g; **Fat:** 14 g (9 of which are monounsaturated); **Vitamin E:** 48% of the daily value (DV); **Manganese:** 27% of the DV; **Magnesium:** 18% of the DV; a decent amount of copper, vitamin B2 (riboflavin), and phosphorus

This is all from a small handful of almonds, which has 164 calories and 6 grams of carbohydrates, which includes 3.5 grams of fiber.

It is important to note that your body does not absorb about 6% of the fats in almonds because this fat is inaccessible to digestive enzymes.

Almonds are also high in phytic acid, a substance that binds certain minerals and prevents them from being absorbed by the body.

While phytic acid is generally considered a healthy antioxidant, it also slightly reduces the amount of iron, zinc, and calcium your body absorbs from almonds.

Summary: Almonds are very popular tree nuts. They are high in healthy monounsaturated fats, fibre, protein, and various important nutrients.

2. Almonds are loaded with antioxidants

Almonds are a fantastic source of antioxidants.

Antioxidants help protect against oxidative stress, which can damage molecules in your cells and contribute to inflammation, aging, and diseases like cancer.

The powerful antioxidants in almonds are largely concentrated in the brown layer of their skin.

For this reason, blanched almonds — those with skin removed — have less antioxidant capacity. This means they may not offer the same anti-inflammatory capabilities.

A 2022 analysis of 16 clinical trials including over 800 participants found that eating up to 60 g (about 2.25 oz) of almonds per day reduced two different markers of inflammation in the body.

These findings support those of another study, which found that eating 2 oz (56 g) of almonds daily for 12 weeks reduced markers of inflammation among a group of over 200 participants between ages 16 and 25.

Summary: Almonds are high in antioxidants that can protect your cells from oxidative damage, a major contributor to aging and disease.

3. Almonds are high in vitamin E

Vitamin E is a family of fat-soluble antioxidants.

These antioxidants are found within the structure of cell membranes in your body, protecting your cells from oxidative damage.

Almonds are among the world's best sources of vitamin E. Just 1 oz provides 48% of the DV.

Several studies have linked higher vitamin E intake with lower rates of heart disease, cancer, and Alzheimer's disease. However, more research is needed to fully confirm these benefits.

Summary: Almonds are among the world's best sources of vitamin E. Getting plenty of vitamin E from foods is linked to numerous health benefits.

4. Almonds can assist with blood sugar control

Nuts are low in carbs but high in healthy fats, protein, and fibre.

This makes them a perfect choice for people with diabetes.

Another boon of almonds is their remarkably high amount of magnesium.

Magnesium is a mineral involved in more than 300 bodily processes, including blood sugar management.

The daily value for magnesium is 420 milligrams (mg). And 2 oz of almonds provides almost half that amount: 153 mg of this important mineral.

Interestingly, it is estimated that at least a quarter of people with type 2 diabetes have a deficiency in magnesium. Adequate magnesium intake has been associated with a reduced risk of type 2 diabetes and improved blood sugar management in people with diabetes.

Magnesium may also be linked to reductions in insulin resistance among people with and without diabetes.

This indicates that foods high in magnesium, such as almonds, may help prevent metabolic syndrome and type 2 diabetes, both of which are major health concerns.

Summary: Almonds are extremely high in magnesium, a mineral that many people don't get enough of. High magnesium intake may offer major improvements for metabolic syndrome and type 2 diabetes.

5. Magnesium also benefits blood pressure levels

The magnesium in almonds may also help lower blood pressure levels.

High blood pressure is one of the leading drivers of heart attacks, strokes, and kidney failure.

A deficiency in magnesium is strongly linked to high blood pressure.

Several meta-analyses have suggested that magnesium supplementation can significantly lower blood pressure among people with and without high blood pressure, as well as people with preexisting chronic disease.

Adding one to two servings of almonds to your diet can help you meet the recommended daily magnesium intake, which may have positive effects on your health.

Summary: Low magnesium levels are strongly linked to high blood pressure, indicating that almonds can help manage blood pressure.

6. Almonds can lower cholesterol levels

High levels of low-density lipoproteins (LDLs) in your blood — also known as "bad" cholesterol — are a well-known risk factor for heart disease.

Your diet can have major effects on LDL levels. Some studies have suggested almonds may be effective in lowering LDL.

A 6-week study including 107 participants at high risk of cardiovascular disease found that a diet providing 20% of calories from almonds lowered LDL cholesterol levels by an average of 9.7 milligrams per deciliter (mg/dL).

Another study found that eating 1.5 oz (42 g) of almonds per day lowered LDL cholesterol by 5.3 mg/dL while maintaining high-density lipoproteins (HDLs), or "good" cholesterol. Participants also lost belly fat.

Summary: Eating one or two handfuls of almonds per day can lead to mild reductions in LDL (bad) cholesterol, potentially reducing the risk of heart disease.

7. Almonds prevent harmful oxidation of LDL cholesterol

Almonds do more than just lower LDL levels in your blood.

They also protect LDL from oxidation, which is a crucial step in the development of atherosclerosis. Atherosclerosis is the narrowing of arteries caused by fatty plaque buildup on the artery wall lining, which increases the risk of heart disease.

Almond skin is rich in polyphenol antioxidants, which prevent the oxidation of cholesterol in test-tube and animal studies).

The effect may be even stronger when combined with other antioxidants such as vitamin E.

One human study including 27 participants showed that snacking on almonds for 1 month lowered oxidized LDL cholesterol levels by 14%.

This may lead to a reduced risk of heart disease over time. More research, including larger human studies, is needed to confirm this.

Summary: LDL (bad) cholesterol can become oxidized, which is a crucial step in the development of atherosclerosis. Snacking on almonds may significantly reduce oxidized LDL.

8. Eating almonds reduces hunger

Almonds are high in protein and fibre.

Both protein and fibre are known to increase feelings of fullness. This can help prevent you from overeating.

One 4-week study in 137 participants showed that a daily 1.5-oz (43-g) serving of almonds significantly reduced hunger and the desire to ea.

Numerous other studies support the hunger-fighting effects of nuts.

Summary: Nuts are high in protein and fibre. Studies show that eating almonds and other nuts can increase fullness and help prevent overeating.

9. Almonds may be effective for weight loss

Nuts contain several nutrients that your body struggles to break down and digest.

Your body does not absorb about 6% of the calories in nuts. Additionally, some evidence suggests that eating nuts can boost metabolism slightly.

Due to their satiating properties, nuts are a great addition to an effective weight loss diet.

Quality human research supports this.

A review of 64 clinical trials and 14 meta-analyses reported that almonds were the only nut that showed a small but significant reduction in body weight and fat mass.

Another study including 100 overweight women found that those consuming almonds lost more weight than those on a nut-free diet. They also showed improvements in waist circumference and other health markers.

It should be noted that both this study and the one above required participants to follow low calorie diets in addition to eating almonds.

Despite being high in fat, almonds are definitely a weight-loss-friendly food.

Almonds and other nuts are very high in calories. So, it is important to be mindful when snacking on almonds and other nuts. As with all foods, moderation is key.

Summary: Though almonds are high in calories, eating them doesn't seem to promote weight gain. Some studies even suggest the opposite, showing that almonds can enhance weight loss.

The bottom line

Given that almonds are a tree nut, which is one of the 9 most common allergens, it may be important to avoid almonds if you are allergic to them.

It's important to note that most current studies have focused on the effects of raw almonds as opposed to other almond products. More research is needed in this area.

Almonds contain lots of healthy fats, fibre, protein, magnesium, and vitamin E.

The health benefits of almonds include lower blood sugar levels, reduced blood pressure, and lower cholesterol levels. They can also reduce hunger and promote weight loss.

Overall, almonds are as close to perfect as a food can get, with some considerations.

www.ingramcontent.com/pod-product-compliance
Ingram Content Group UK Ltd.
Pitfield, Milton Keynes, MK11 3LW, UK
UKHW020243240426
12048UKWH00026B/1587